PumpOne®

SWISS
BALL

FOR CORE STRENGTH

DECLAN CONDRON

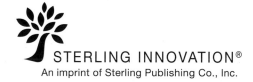

STERLING INNOVATION®
An imprint of Sterling Publishing Co., Inc.

New York / London
www.sterlingpublishing.com

STERLING and the distinctive Sterling logo are registered trademarks of Sterling Publishing Co., Inc.

Library of Congress Cataloging-in-Publication Data

Condron, Declan.
  Swiss ball for core strength / Declan Condron.
     p. cm. -- (Health series)
  Includes index.
  ISBN 978-1-4027-5971-0
  1. Swiss exercise balls. 2. Exercise. I. Title.
  GV484.C663 2008
  613.7'10284--dc22

                         2008018550

10 9 8 7 6 5 4 3 2 1

Published by Sterling Publishing Co., Inc.
387 Park Avenue South, New York, NY 10016
© 2008 by PumpOne®
Distributed in Canada by Sterling Publishing
c/o Canadian Manda Group, 165 Dufferin Street
Toronto, Ontario, Canada M6K 3H6
Distributed in the United Kingdom by GMC Distribution Services
Castle Place, 166 High Street, Lewes, East Sussex, England BN7 1XU
Distributed in Australia by Capricorn Link (Australia) Pty. Ltd.
P.O. Box 704, Windsor, NSW 2756, Australia

Digital Imaging by Craig Schlossberg
Photography by Susan E. Cohen

Sterling ISBN 978-1-4027-5971-0

For information about custom editions, special sales, premium and corporate purchases, please contact
Sterling Special Sales Department at 800-805-5489 or specialsales@sterlingpublishing.com.

The exercise programs described in this book are based on well-established practices proven to be effective for overall health and fitness, but they are not a substitute for personalized advice from a qualified practitioner. Always consult with a qualified health care professional in matters relating to your health before beginning this or any exercise program. This is especially important if you are pregnant or nursing, if you are elderly, or if you have any chronic or recurring medical condition. As with any exercise program, if at any point during your workout you begin to feel faint, dizzy, or have physical discomfort, you should stop immediately and consult a physician.

The purpose of this book is to educate and is sold with the understanding that the author and the publisher shall have neither liability nor responsibility for any injury caused or alleged to be caused directly or indirectly by the information in this book.

CONTENTS

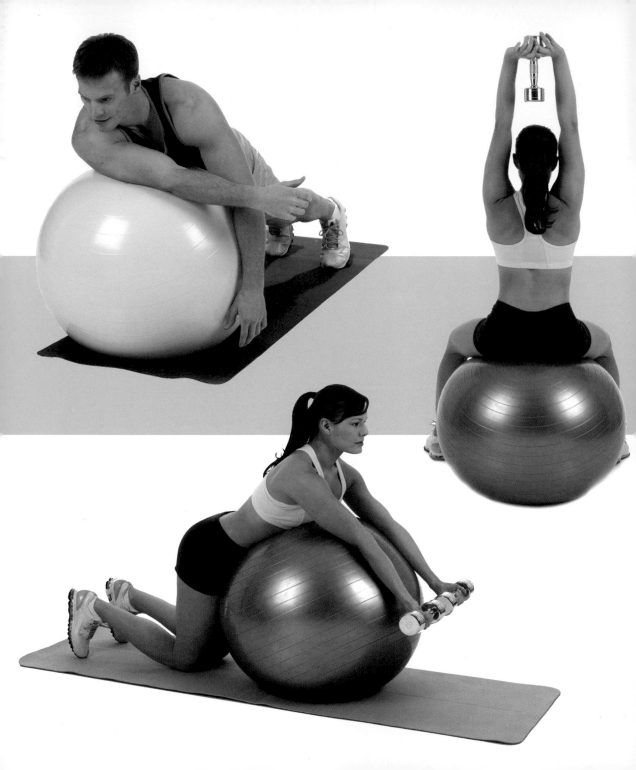

INTRODUCTION

Welcome to *Swiss Ball for Core Strength*. This book is designed to provide multiple workouts using a Swiss ball, some light dumbbells, ankle weights, and a mat. These workouts can be done anywhere: at home, while traveling, or at the gym. (Most gyms will have all the necessary equipment.)

Using a Swiss ball for exercise is not a new concept. The ball has been a part of rehabilitation and physical therapy for many years. It was first introduced in Switzerland in 1963, thus the name "Swiss ball." (Some people call it a gymnastic ball or a fit ball.) Swiss balls gained popularity in gyms and health clubs in the 1990s and are now standard equipment in most exercise facilities.

This book on Swiss ball core training is not just a list of exercises. It provides specific, graduated workouts. The workouts are divided into three levels, with four workouts each, and each level gets progressively more challenging. Use this book as a guide to proper form for the individual exercises as you reach each new workout level.

SO WHAT'S THE BIG DEAL WITH THE BALL?

Why use a Swiss ball? It looks slippery and unstable. Might be a little dangerous? What can it do for you? Swiss balls are completely safe and offer many benefits for fitness training. Actually, it's the very instability of a Swiss ball that makes it such an excellent exercise tool. Just by sitting on the ball, you activate the stabilizer muscles of your core.

BENEFITS OF A REGULAR SWISS BALL EXERCISE PROGRAM

INCREASED NEUROMUSCULAR FUNCTIONING

The neuromuscular system forms the connections among the brain, central nervous system, and the muscles. To perform a movement or action, your brain sends a message via the nervous system to the muscles to go into action. Using a Swiss ball involves greater muscle activity and ignites more and better-quality messages moving through the nerve–muscle conduit from the brain.

IMPROVEMENTS IN COORDINATION AND PROPRIOCEPTION

As the brain communicates with the muscles, the muscles talk back to the brain. This phenomenon is called proprioception, and sometimes kinesthesia. Muscles sense where your limbs are in space, and they send a signal to your brain: "Your left arm is above your head," or "Your right leg is straight out in front." A Swiss ball challenges proprioception because it is less stable than a bench and requires quick adjustment to maintain balance. That messaging between the brain and muscles builds better coordination and proprioception.

DEVELOP BETTER MUSCLE SYNERGY

Contrary to popular belief, a muscle group does not work by itself. Muscle groups work together to facilitate movement, and also to stabilize and support inert body parts. For example, during a biceps curl, your biceps muscles contract to move your arm, while your deltoid muscles help the movement and also stabilize your shoulder. Meanwhile, the triceps work to control the speed of the movement. Using a Swiss ball can help develop better synergy among muscle groups.

VARIETY

Our bodies are very smart machines. When our bodies ask us to move, our brain figures out the easiest way to do it. A body asked to perform a movement again and again finds the effort becomes increasingly easy. Changing the task slightly gives our bodies a new challenge: to figure out a better way to meet new requirements. A Swiss ball is a great tool to change a workout and give the body new stimuli.

THE CORE DEFINED

Our body's core is commonly defined as the deep abdominal and spinal muscles that support the spine and help to maintain a neutral position during movement. That description is partly true. The definition of the core can be expanded to include almost all the muscles of the torso. It includes the smaller deep muscles, such as the *transverse abdominus* and *multifidius*, but also the larger muscles such as the *rectus abdominus*, *quadratus lumborum* (lower back muscles that maintain spinal and pelvic balance), internal and external obliques, the *erector spinae*, the *latissimus dorsi* and *ilio-psoas* muscles.

This muscular core acts like a corset that can stabilize, move, resist movement, and lend support all at once. Remember, muscle groups don't act in isolation; they act in synergy to produce the best movement strategy possible. Therefore, core muscles work together to produce the most efficient movement, but not always the safest movement.

THE SWISS BALL AND THE BACK

Back pain is one of the most common physical ailments in the United States today. It is estimated that eight out of ten people will suffer some form of back pain at some stage in their life. Those statistics are not very encouraging, but there is hope: With a good overall fitness lifestyle, we can greatly reduce that risk. Originally the Swiss ball was used to rehabilitate adults with orthopedic injuries, including back injuries. Any of us can go a long way in keeping our backs strong, healthy, and free of injury by using a Swiss ball to strengthen core muscle groups, increase their neuromuscular functioning, improve their proprioception and coordination, and develop overall muscle synergy.

A WORD ABOUT POSTURE

Posture can be defined as the position or bearing of the body. It refers to the overall alignment of body parts to each other when one is standing in a relaxed position. Posture is the result of many processes and tensions in the body. It becomes a measure of overall balance. With good posture, a person's overall structure is in good mechanical balance. Bad posture is the result when some areas of the body don't permit the appropriate mechanical ability. Poor posture can lead to mechanical problems, dysfunctions, and pain.

Let's take a look at the spine. If a person can position his spine so his vertebrae are aligned over one another without lateral curvature, and his muscles, ligaments, and tendons balance his weight with minimal effort, he is in a good neutral spinal posture with respect to the force of gravity. If, however, one vertebra is off track, or one muscle is not functioning, alignment is off and can cause excessive stress on the spine, resulting in injury. Exercise, stretching, massage, and careful training can help to restore balance and good posture. A Swiss ball is an excellent training stimulus. In these workouts, you will see the phrase "maintain a neutral spine." This suggestion refers to having good posture throughout the spine, having everything aligned naturally with all the soft tissues—muscles, tendons, ligaments, and nerves—remaining strong.

HOW THIS BOOK WORKS

This book is organized to provide a progressive exercise plan. Like a personal trainer, it is a guide to what exercises to perform, in which order, and when to advance to a new level to keep you working toward a stronger, fitter body.

The book is divided into three difficulty levels, each containing four workouts. Every workout contains ten different exercises. Workouts can be performed at different intensities, by varying the number of repetitions and sets, the load used, and the amount of rest between sets. Some exercises work one side at a time; do these on both sides for the full repetitions. The book offers two different intensity tracks for each workout: the toning track and the weight-loss track. The toning track concentrates on building strength and defining muscles; the weight-loss track concentrates on losing weight. There is some crossover between tracks: If you are on the weight-loss track, you will also see increases in muscle strength and definition; on the toning track, you might also lose weight.

The three levels provide an exercise plan that becomes more difficult as you get fitter.

We suggest beginning at level one and working your way up to level three, even if you are already experienced with workouts. Level-three workouts can be very challenging and may take some time to master, so don't rush yourself—enjoy the journey.

Whether you choose the toning or weight-loss track, try to do two to three workout sessions per week. Just as the body needs variety, it also needs consistency. Perform each workout a few times in each level before moving forward. Spend a number of weeks rotating through the workouts in level one before attempting levels two and three.

A PLAN FOR TOTAL HEALTH

Before you reach for your Swiss ball, take a few minutes to consider the whole picture. Exercising with a Swiss ball should be part of a plan for total health, a plan that takes some dedication and hard work. No one gets fit and strong overnight. Using a Swiss ball is a great tool for achieving strength and fitness, but it is not a cure-all. An overall health plan should incorporate a number of practices and habits that have an impact on your body. There are five essentials components to a health plan—strength training; cardiovascular training; flexibility and mobility; a healthy nutrition plan; and adequate rest and recovery. An effective Swiss ball exercise program depends on all five of these measures. The right emphasis on each depends on your individual goal.

SAFETY PRECAUTIONS

As with any exercise program, safety is of the utmost importance for Swiss ball training. The last thing you want to do is to injure yourself trying to get into better shape and improve your health. Before you start, we recommend you do the following:

TALK TO YOUR DOCTOR

Always consult your doctor before starting a fitness program, especially if you have or have had a chronic medical condition, are taking any medications, or are pregnant.

Immediately stop exercising if you feel pain, faintness, dizziness, or shortness of breath. Wait awhile. You may decide to quit for the day, or resume slowly.

GET EQUIPPED

Check the condition of the Swiss ball and any other equipment. Make sure you choose the right ball for your body size. Follow the manufacturer's instructions for inflation.

Read all warnings and instructions on the proper use and maintenance of all equipment before you begin.

MAKE ROOM

Make sure you have enough space in which to exercise, and avoid exercising on slippery surfaces. Be aware of the surrounding areas, other people, and any obstacles that might cause a fall.

SUIT UP

Wear appropriate exercise clothing that is neither too baggy nor too tight. Also be sure to put on some form of footwear. Sneakers are comfortable and have a nonslip sole.

WARM UP AND COOL DOWN

Always warm up for at least five minutes before starting any workout. Warming up gets the body ready to exercise and increases its core temperature and muscle elasticity. We have provided some warm-up tips a little later in the book. Also be sure to cool down and stretch after your workout. Doing so will help relax your muscles and return them to their resting length, and reduce to normal your core temperature.

HAVE WATER ON HAND

It's a good idea to eat something at least two hours before exercising, and always to have water on hand while you are working out. Right after working out is a great time to replenish the body's energy supplies, while you relax and rest.

EQUIPMENT

The workouts in this book require the use of the following equipment:

SWISS BALL

It wouldn't be much of a Swiss ball exercise program without a Swiss ball. They come in various sizes and colors. Be sure to choose the correct ball for you. Manufacturers provide size guidelines based on height. A general rule of thumb is that when you are seated on the ball, your hips should be slightly higher than your knees, and your feet should be flat on the floor.

The following size chart can also be used as a general rule.

BALL SIZE GUIDELINES FOR EXERCISE	
HEIGHT	**BALL SIZE**
Under 5'2" (1.57 m)	45 cm
5'3"–5'8" (1.60 m–1.72 m)	55 cm
5'9"–6'2" (1.75 m–1.88 m)	65 cm
Above 6'3" (1.90 m)	75 cm

Inflate the ball according to the manufacturer's guidelines. Most balls come with a hand or foot pump.

DUMBBELLS

Weighted dumbbells come in many shapes and sizes and many appealing colors. Since you will be using different muscle groups, some bigger and stronger than others, we recommend having a selection of sizes. A range from 5 to15 pounds should be sufficient at first. You can always add more weight as you gain strength and tone your muscles.

ANKLE WEIGHTS

Ankle weights are great for adding resistance to exercises for the lower limbs. We recommend the wraparound type with adjustable weight inserts, easily removed or replaced when necessary.

EXERCISE MAT

Some of our exercises require you to lie on the floor. It's a good idea to work on a basic yoga or Pilates mat rather than the floor. The mat will also provide a nonslip surface during other exercises.

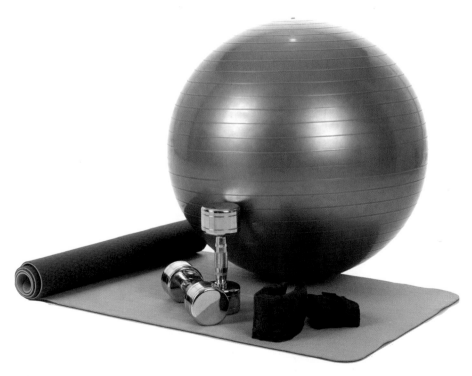

GETTING STARTED

Ready to get started? You have your equipment and are eager to perform those first repetitions. Consider a few last tips before you begin. If this is your first time using a Swiss ball or if it's been a while, take some time to get familiar with sitting and lying and eventually kneeling on it. Take it easy at first. Practice these three positions.

SIT ON THE BALL

Sit on the top center of the ball with your feet flat on the floor. Your hips should be slightly higher than your knees. Keep your head up and look straight ahead, aligning your shoulders over your hips. Be conscious of the position of your spine at all times. Do not let your shoulders roll forward, and don't flex your lower back. Awareness of your form will help you establish good posture along your spine while seated on the ball.

LIE ON THE BALL

Lie facedown with the ball under your midsection and your hands and feet on the floor. Practice rolling forward and backward, lifting your hands or feet as you roll. Once you feel comfortable with those movements, move side to side, and work up to lying on the ball without your hands or feet touching the floor.

Next, turn over on your back and center the ball between your shoulder blades. Place your feet flat on the floor and your hands on your hips. Keep your hips level with your shoulders. This is known as the reverse bridge position. It requires you to contract your abdominal and core muscles and will be used a lot in the exercises.

KNEEL ON THE BALL

For this position, keep something sturdy like a chair or a bench close by to help with balance. Place both hands and one knee on top of the ball. Slowly lift your other leg off the floor, and place your other knee on the ball. You should now be on all fours atop the ball. Now place one hand on the chair to help stabilize you, and lift the other hand off the ball. Move your upper body upright. Just as with the seated position, you should be conscious of the position of your spine. Do not let your shoulders roll forward, or flex your lower back. Take your hand off the support, and practice holding your body upright. You will move around some, so try to relax and find your center of balance.

Once you are comfortable with these positions on the ball, you are ready to start working out. Be sure to concentrate on your breathing as you perform the exercises. Whether you breathe in or out as you lift the dumbbells is not so important as remembering to breathe. Do not hold your breath.

WARMING UP AND COOLING DOWN

A warm-up is a crucial part of any exercise program. The importance of a structured warm-up cannot be overstated. It is essential for getting the body ready for activity and helping to prevent injury. Warming up before working out prepares you for strenuous activity by increasing the temperatures of both the body's core and muscles. Increasing the temperature of your muscles helps to loosen them, making them more supple and flexible.

Warming up also increases your heart rate and the rate of your blood flow to your muscles, thereby increasing the delivery of oxygen and nutrients to them and helping prepare them and other tissues for activity.

A concise warm-up should last 10 to 15 minutes. It should target all areas of the body, starting with gentle activity, such as light cardiovascular work. It should gradually increase in intensity, building up to movements similar to the exercises in the workout. Static stretching before working out is optional.

Just as important as warming up before exercising is a good cool-down afterward. Cooling down helps return your core temperature to normal and helps muscles relax and return to their original length. Static stretching during a cool-down can help to increase muscle and joint range of motion, which will improve flexibility and may reduce muscle soreness.

SQUAT TO BALL OVERHEAD

- Start in a squat position, with your feet flat and your back in a neutral position. Hold the ball out in front of you at waist height.

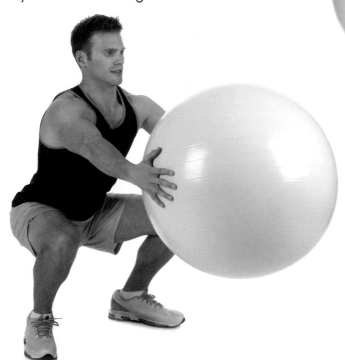

- Stand tall and raise the ball overhead, extending your arms fully.

- Perform 10 to 15 repetitions. Be sure to squat as low as you can and to stretch as high as you can.

OVERHEAD CIRCLES

- Hold the ball overhead, with your arms fully extended.

- Make a big circle overhead with the ball, moving through your midsection.

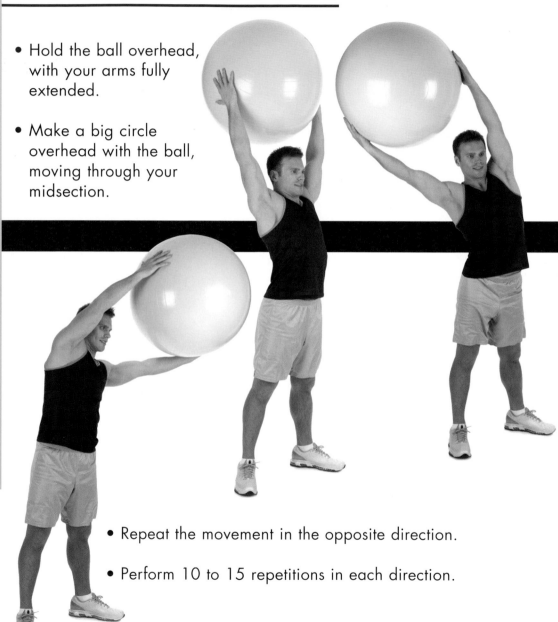

- Repeat the movement in the opposite direction.

- Perform 10 to 15 repetitions in each direction.

SIDE ROTATIONS

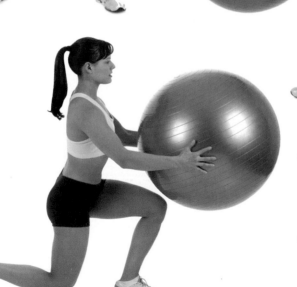

- Stand upright, holding the ball at waist height.

- Rotate to one side, bending your hips and knees and lowering your body toward the floor.

- Switch sides, holding the ball at waist height throughout.

- Keep your head up and look straight ahead to maintain a neutral spine. Perform 10 to 15 repetitions in both directions.

SEATED TRUNK ROTATIONS

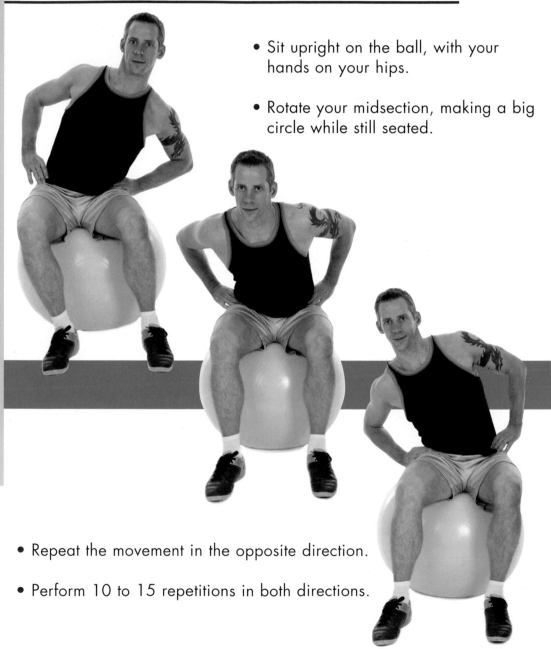

- Sit upright on the ball, with your hands on your hips.

- Rotate your midsection, making a big circle while still seated.

- Repeat the movement in the opposite direction.

- Perform 10 to 15 repetitions in both directions.

#1 DEADLIFT

- Start in a squat position, with your feet flat on the floor, head up, and back in a neutral position.

- Hold the ball on the floor in front of you.

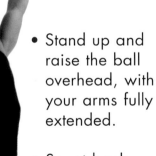

HINTS

• In squatting exercises, the back position is very important. Always maintain a neutral position; do not round your lower back or overarch it. • Keep your head up, looking straight forward and your shoulders back.

STRENGTH INTENSITY	TONE INTENSITY
3 sets	2 sets
15 reps	20 reps
45 seconds rest between sets	30 seconds rest between sets

- Stand up and raise the ball overhead, with your arms fully extended.

- Squat back down, returning to the starting position with the ball on the floor in front.

#2 CHEST PRESS

- Lie on your back on the ball in a reverse bridge position, with the ball between your shoulder blades.

- Keep your hips level with your shoulders and your feet flat on the floor.

- Hold a dumbbell in each hand at shoulder level.

- Press the dumbbells up until your arms are straight and the dumbbells are directly over your upper chest.

- Lower the dumbbells by bending at the elbows and returning to the starting position.

- Make sure to go all the way down till the dumbbells are back to shoulder level.

STRENGTH INTENSITY	TONE INTENSITY
3 sets	2 sets
15 reps	20 reps
45 seconds rest between sets	30 seconds rest between sets

HINTS

- Keep your hips in line with your shoulders; do not let them sag or dip.
- Keep the dumbbell directly over the chest. • Start with your feet about shoulder-width apart.

#3 UPRIGHT ROW

- Sit upright on the ball, with your feet flat on the floor.

- Hold a dumbbell in each hand, with your palms facing backward and your arms extended by your sides.

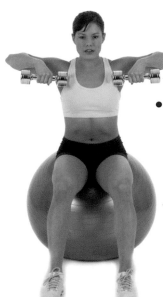

- Raise the dumbbells up in front under your chin, bringing the elbows above your shoulders.

- Lower the dumbbells to the starting position at your sides.

STRENGTH INTENSITY	TONE INTENSITY
3 sets	2 sets
15 reps	20 reps
45 seconds rest between sets	30 seconds rest between sets

HINTS

• When raising the dumbbells, make sure to bring your elbows higher than your shoulders at the top. • Do not turn your wrists; keep the dumbbells level throughout the movement.

#4 WIDE ROW

- Lie facedown on the ball, with it under your mid-abdomen and your legs stretched out behind.

- Hold a dumbbell in each hand, with your arms extended to the sides of the ball and your elbows slightly bent and sticking out to the sides. Have your palms facing back to the ball.

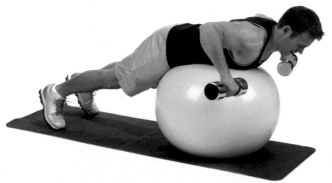

- Raise the dumbbells up, drawing your shoulder blades together and bending your elbows outward.

- Lower the dumbbells back toward the floor, extending at the elbows.

STRENGTH INTENSITY	TONE INTENSITY
3 sets	2 sets
15 reps	20 reps
45 seconds rest between sets	30 seconds rest between sets

HINTS

• Start with your feet about shoulder-width apart. • For the wide row, draw your elbows up and out to your sides—not in close. • Look down at the floor to keep your head in line with your spine.

#5 LEG CURL

- Using ankle weights, start by lying facedown with the ball under your upper legs.

- Place your hands on the mat directly under your shoulders, with your arms fully extended.

- Your body should be in a straight line from head to feet.

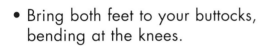

- Bring both feet to your buttocks, bending at the knees.

- Extend your legs, lowering your feet back to the starting position.

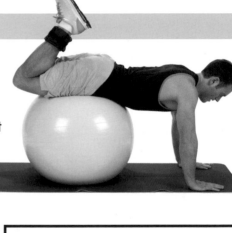

STRENGTH INTENSITY	TONE INTENSITY
3 sets	2 sets
15 reps	20 reps
45 seconds rest between sets	30 seconds rest between sets

HINTS

• To maintain a neutral spine, look at the floor and do not raise your head during the exercise. • Keep your arms fully extended throughout the movement. • Bring your feet all the way in to touch the buttocks and all the way back out to a straight-leg position.

#6 CURL

- Sit upright on the ball, with your feet flat on the floor.

- Hold a dumbbell in each hand, with your palms facing forward and your arms extended by your sides.

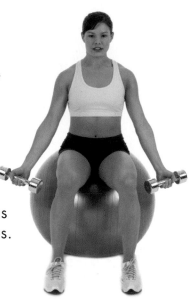

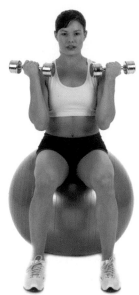

HINTS

• Keep your back upright by contracting your core muscles. Do not round your lower back. • Go through the full range of motion, from arms fully extended to dumbbells at shoulder level and back again.

- Raise the dumbbells up in front to shoulder level, bending at the elbows, and with your palms facing back.

- Lower the dumbbells by straightening your elbows and returning to the starting position.

- Make sure to go all the way down till the arms are fully extended.

STRENGTH INTENSITY	TONE INTENSITY
3 sets	2 sets
15 reps	20 reps
45 seconds rest between sets	30 seconds rest between sets

#7 UNI TRICEPS EXTENSION

- Sit upright on the ball, with your feet flat on the floor.

- Hold a dumbbell in one hand behind your head, with your elbow bent and pointing up.

- Lift the dumbbell up by extending your elbow and straightening your arm directly overhead.

- Lower the dumbbell by bending at the elbow, returning to the starting position behind your head.

- Repeat on the other arm.

STRENGTH INTENSITY	TONE INTENSITY
3 sets	2 sets
15 reps	20 reps
45 seconds rest between sets	30 seconds rest between sets

HINTS

• Keep your back upright by contracting your core muscles; do not round your lower back. • Be careful not to bang the dumbbell against the back of your head as you lift and lower it. • Go through the full range of motion, from behind the head to the arm fully extended overhead and back again. • Keep your shoulder steady; movement should occur only at the elbow.

#8 BALL CRUNCH

- Lie on your back on the ball in a reverse bridge position, with the ball in the middle of your back. Place your hands to the sides of your head.

- Keep your head and neck off the ball and your feet flat on the ground.

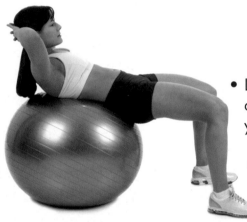

- Lift your head and shoulders up and away from the ball by contracting your abdominals.

- Roll your upper body back over the ball, returning to the starting position.

STRENGTH INTENSITY	TONE INTENSITY
3 sets	2 sets
15 reps	20 reps
45 seconds rest between sets	30 seconds rest between sets

HINTS

• Make sure to control the movement through your midsection and avoid jerky motions. • You should not use your hands to pull your head and neck up. • Lift only your head and shoulders off the ball.

#9 KNEELING OBLIQUE CRUNCH

- Lie on one side on the ball, with one knee on the mat and the other leg stretched out.

- Place your hands to the sides of your head.

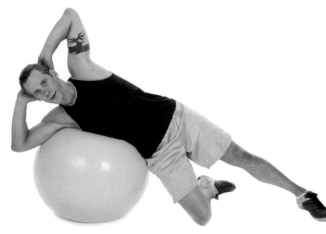

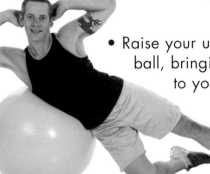

- Raise your upper body up and off the ball, bringing your outside elbow down to your side.

- Lower your body back down, returning to the starting position, lying over the ball.

- Repeat on the other side.

STRENGTH INTENSITY	TONE INTENSITY
3 sets	2 sets
15 reps	20 reps
45 seconds rest between sets	30 seconds rest between sets

HINTS

- Make sure to control the movement through your midsection and avoid jerky motions. • Keep your upper body upright, and do not allow your shoulders to fall forward or your elbows to come together.

#10 TWISTING CRUNCH

- Lie on your back on the ball in a reverse bridge position, with the ball in the middle of your back.

- Keep your head and neck off the ball and your feet flat on the ground.

- Place your hands to the sides of your head.

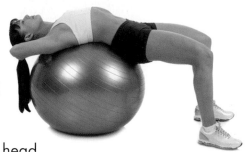

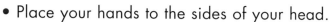

- Lift your head and shoulders up and away from the ball and rotate them to one side by contracting your abdominals and twisting through the midsection.

- Twist back to the center, and roll your upper body back over the ball, returning to the starting position.

- Repeat in the other direction.

STRENGTH INTENSITY	TONE INTENSITY
3 sets	2 sets
15 reps	20 reps
45 seconds rest between sets	30 seconds rest between sets

HINTS

- Make sure to control the movement through your midsection and avoid jerky motions. • You should not use your hands to pull your head and neck up; lift only your head and shoulders up off the ball, not your whole back.

#1 SQUAT TO BALL

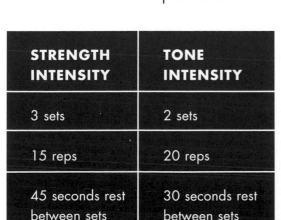

- Start with the ball on the floor a little behind you.

- Standing upright with a dumbbell in each hand, place your feet facing forward, about hip-width apart.

- Lower your body down to the ball till you just touch it.

- Keep your back in a neutral position.

- Push through the feet to return to the starting position.

STRENGTH INTENSITY	TONE INTENSITY
3 sets	2 sets
15 reps	20 reps
45 seconds rest between sets	30 seconds rest between sets

HINTS

- In squatting exercises, the back position is very important. Maintain a neutral position, and do not round your lower back. • Keep your head up, looking straight forward, and your shoulders back.

#2 CLOSE ROW

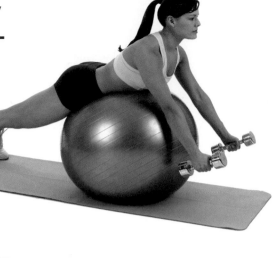

- Lie facedown on the ball, with it under your mid-abdomen and your legs stretched out behind.

- Hold a dumbbell in each hand, with your arms extended at the sides of the ball and your elbows slightly bent, palms facing each other.

- Raise the dumbbells up by drawing your shoulder blades together and bending your elbows.

- Lower the dumbbells back toward the floor to the starting position, extending at the elbows.

STRENGTH INTENSITY	TONE INTENSITY
3 sets	2 sets
15 reps	20 reps
45 seconds rest between sets	30 seconds rest between sets

HINTS

- Start with your feet about shoulder-width apart. • Draw your elbows up by your sides, not outward. • Look down at the floor to keep your head in line with your spine.

#3 DUMBBELL PULLOVER

- Lie on your back in a reverse bridge position, with the ball between your shoulder blades and feet flat on the floor. Keep your hips level with your shoulders.

- Hold one dumbbell in both hands, with your arms fully extended upward and the dumbbell directly over your chest.

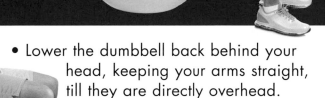

- Lower the dumbbell back behind your head, keeping your arms straight, till they are directly overhead.

- Return the dumbbell to the starting position over your chest.

- Keep your arms completely straight throughout the movement.

STRENGTH INTENSITY	TONE INTENSITY
3 sets	2 sets
15 reps	20 reps
45 seconds rest between sets	30 seconds rest between sets

HINTS

- Keep your hips in line with your shoulders; do not let them sag or dip.
- You can lower the dumbbell farther behind your head once you feel comfortable with the movement.

#4 LATERAL RAISE

- Sit upright on the ball with your feet flat on the floor.

- Hold a dumbbell in each hand, with your palms facing in and your arms extended by your sides.

HINTS

- Keep your back upright by contracting your core muscles as you raise the dumbbells up to the sides. • Avoid jerky movements. • You can bend the elbows slightly to avoid too much stress on the shoulder joint.

STRENGTH INTENSITY	TONE INTENSITY
3 sets	2 sets
15 reps	20 reps
45 seconds rest between sets	30 seconds rest between sets

- Raise the dumbbells up and out to the sides, going just above shoulder level and keeping your arms straight.

- Lower the dumbbells back down to your sides, returning to the starting position.

- Make sure to go all the way down till the arms are fully extended.

#5 FLAT FLY

- Lie on your back in a reverse bridge position, with the ball between your shoulder blades. Keep your hips level with your shoulders.

- Hold a dumbbell in each hand, with your arms fully extended overhead and your palms facing in. Keep a slight bend in the elbows throughout.

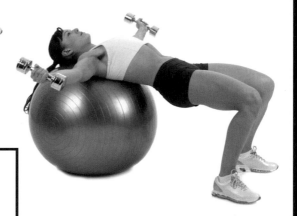

HINT

- Keep your hips in line with your shoulders; do not let them sag or dip.

- Lower the dumbbells out to the sides and down to shoulder level.

- Return to your starting position, coming all the way back to a fully extended position overhead.

STRENGTH INTENSITY	TONE INTENSITY
3 sets	2 sets
15 reps	20 reps
45 seconds rest between sets	30 seconds rest between sets

#6 HAMMER CURL

- Sit upright on the ball, with your feet flat on the floor.

- Hold a dumbbell in each hand, with your palms facing in and your arms extended by your sides.

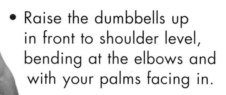

- Raise the dumbbells up in front to shoulder level, bending at the elbows and with your palms facing in.

- Lower the dumbbells by straightening your elbows and returning to the starting position. Make sure to go all the way down till your arms are fully extended.

STRENGTH INTENSITY	TONE INTENSITY
3 sets	2 sets
15 reps	20 reps
45 seconds rest between sets	30 seconds rest between sets

HINTS

• Keep your back upright by contracting your core muscles. Do not round your lower back. • Go through the full range of motion, from arms fully extended to dumbbells at shoulder level and back again.

#7 TRICEPS EXTENSION

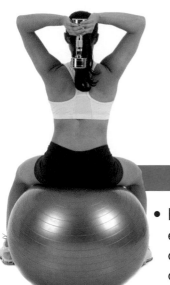

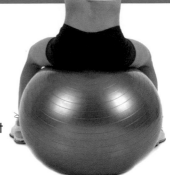

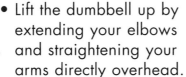

- Sit upright on the ball, with your feet flat on the floor.

- Hold a dumbbell at one end in both hands behind your head, with your elbows bent.

- Lift the dumbbell up by extending your elbows and straightening your arms directly overhead.

- Lower the dumbbell by bending at the elbows, returning to the starting position behind your head.

STRENGTH INTENSITY	TONE INTENSITY
3 sets	2 sets
15 reps	20 reps
45 seconds rest between sets	30 seconds rest between sets

HINTS

• Keep your back upright by contracting your core muscles. Do not round your lower back. • Be careful not to bang the dumbbell against the back of your head as you lift and lower it. • Go through the full range of motion, from behind the head to the arm fully extended overhead and back again. • Keep your shoulders steady; movement should occur only at the elbows.

#8 FEET-UP CRUNCH

- Lie flat, with your back on the mat, knees bent, and your heels on top of the ball. Place your hands to the sides of your head.

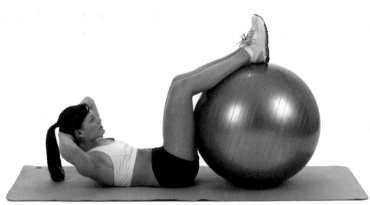

- Lift your head and shoulders off the mat by contracting your abdominals.

- Roll your head and shoulders back to the mat, returning to the starting position.

STRENGTH INTENSITY	TONE INTENSITY
3 sets	2 sets
15 reps	20 reps
45 seconds rest between sets	30 seconds rest between sets

HINTS

- Make sure to control the movement through your midsection, and avoid jerky motions. • You should not use your hands to pull your head and neck up. • Lift only your head and shoulders up off floor, not your whole back.

- Lie on your back on the mat, with your heels on top of the ball.

- Place your hands on the mat by your sides.

- Raise your hips off the mat by contracting your core and abdominal muscles.

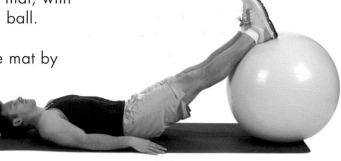

- Hold at the top for 10 seconds; then lower your body back to the mat, returning to the starting position.

STRENGTH INTENSITY	TONE INTENSITY
3 sets	2 sets
15 reps	20 reps
45 seconds rest between sets	30 seconds rest between sets

HINTS

- Keep your core and abdominal muscles contracted, and maintain a neutral spine throughout the movement. • Push your hands into the floor to help stabilize yourself when raising your hips.
- Only your head, upper back, arms, and shoulders should be in contact with the mat at the top position.

#10 LOWER BODY TWIST

- Lie on your back on the mat, legs lifted, with the ball between your bent knees. Place your hands on the mat at your sides.

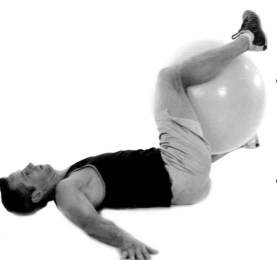

- Rotate your lower body down to one side till your knee touches the floor, keeping the ball between your feet.

- Rotate to the other side 180 degrees, touching the floor with the other knee.

STRENGTH INTENSITY	TONE INTENSITY
3 sets	2 sets
15 reps	20 reps
45 seconds rest between sets	30 seconds rest between sets

HINTS

- Keep your shoulders and upper back on the mat throughout the movement.
- Twist through your midsection, using your abdominal muscles to perform the movement.

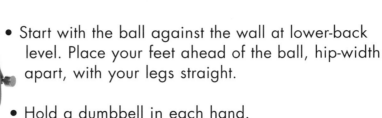

#1 WALL SQUAT

- Start with the ball against the wall at lower-back level. Place your feet ahead of the ball, hip-width apart, with your legs straight.

- Hold a dumbbell in each hand.

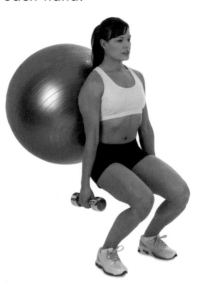

HINTS

• Keep your head up and look straight ahead throughout the movement. Do not look down at the floor or at your feet.
• Make sure to keep your feet flat on the floor, with your heel down as you move up and down. • Keep pushing back against the ball throughout the movement.

STRENGTH INTENSITY	TONE INTENSITY
3 sets	2 sets
15 reps	20 reps
45 seconds rest between sets	30 seconds rest between sets

- Lower your body down toward the floor, pushing back slightly against the ball.

- Stop when your thighs are parallel to the floor.

- Push through your feet to return to the starting position.

#2 BENT-OVER ROW

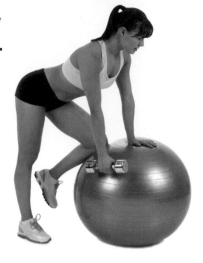

- Place one knee and the same-side hand on the ball.

- Hold a dumbbell in the other hand by your side, with your arm fully extended.

- Place the other foot flat on the floor, a little behind and to the side of the ball.

- Raise the dumbbell up to your chest, bending at the elbow.

- Lower the dumbbell back to the starting position, and keep your back in a neutral position throughout the movement.

- Repeat on the other arm.

STRENGTH INTENSITY	TONE INTENSITY
3 sets	2 sets
15 reps	20 reps
45 seconds rest between sets	30 seconds rest between sets

HINTS

• Look down toward the floor to maintain a neutral spine. • Do not lift your head as you lift the dumbbell. • Raise the dumbbell so that your elbow comes above your shoulder.

#3 OVERHEAD PRESS

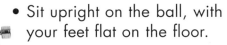

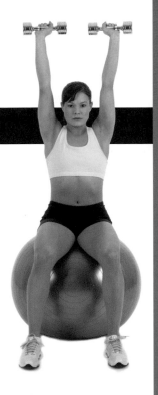

- Sit upright on the ball, with your feet flat on the floor.

- Hold a dumbbell in each hand at shoulder level, with your palms facing forward.

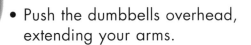

- Push the dumbbells overhead, extending your arms.

- Lower the dumbbells by bending your elbows and returning to the starting position. Make sure to go all the way down till the dumbbells are at your shoulder level.

STRENGTH INTENSITY	TONE INTENSITY
3 sets	2 sets
15 reps	20 reps
45 seconds rest between sets	30 seconds rest between sets

HINTS
• Keep your back upright by contracting your core muscles as you push the dumbbells overhead. Do not round your lower back. • Go through the full range of motion, from shoulder level to arms fully extended overhead and back again.

#4 DUMBBELL INCLINE PRESS

- Lie on your back on the ball in a reverse bridge position, with the ball between your shoulder blades.

- Drop your hips so your back lies on the ball and your body is at a 45-degree angle, with your feet flat on the floor.

- Hold a dumbbell in each hand at shoulder level.

- Press the dumbbells up until your arms are straight and the dumbbells are directly over your upper chest.

- Lower the dumbbells by bending at the elbows and returning to the starting position. Make sure to go all the way down till the dumbbells are back to shoulder level.

STRENGTH INTENSITY	TONE INTENSITY
3 sets	2 sets
15 reps	20 reps
45 seconds rest between sets	30 seconds rest between sets

HINTS

- Although your hips and back are on the ball, keep your abdominal muscles contracted to help keep you stable.
- Keep the dumbbells directly over the chest. Do not let them move outward or inward.

- Kneel on the mat with your forearms on the ball, elbows bent, and your chest nearly touching the ball.

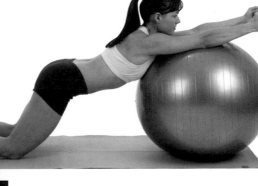

- Push the ball forward, extending your arms and keeping your upper body rigid.

- Pull the ball back, drawing your elbows in until you reach the starting position.

STRENGTH INTENSITY	TONE INTENSITY
3 sets	2 sets
15 reps	20 reps
45 seconds rest between sets	30 seconds rest between sets

HINTS

- Maintain a neutral spine by looking down and not moving your head.
- Make sure to control the movement through your midsection, and avoid jerky motions. • Keep your abdominal and core muscles contracted throughout the movement for stability.

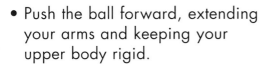

#6 DUMBBELL FRENCH PRESS

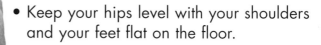

- Lie on your back on the ball in a reverse bridge position, with the ball between your shoulder blades.

- Keep your hips level with your shoulders and your feet flat on the floor.

- Hold a dumbbell in each hand, with your elbows flexed and the weights positioned at the sides of your head (near your ears).

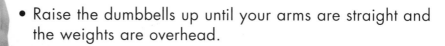

- Raise the dumbbells up until your arms are straight and the weights are overhead.

- Lower the dumbbells, bending at the elbows and returning to the starting position. Make sure to go all the way down till the dumbbells are back at the sides of your head.

STRENGTH INTENSITY	TONE INTENSITY
3 sets	2 sets
15 reps	20 reps
45 seconds rest between sets	30 seconds rest between sets

HINTS

- Keep your hips in line with your shoulders. Do not let them sag or dip.
- Be careful not to bang the dumbbells against your head as you lift and lower them. • Keep the shoulders steady; movement should occur only at the elbows.

#7 TWISTING CURL

- Sit upright on the ball, with your feet flat on the floor.

- Hold a dumbbell in each hand, with your palms facing in and your arms extended by your sides.

- Raise the dumbbells up in front to shoulder level, bending at the elbows and twisting at the wrist to finish with your palms facing back.

- Lower the dumbbells by straightening your elbows and returning to the starting position, with your arms fully extended.

STRENGTH INTENSITY	TONE INTENSITY
3 sets	2 sets
15 reps	20 reps
45 seconds rest between sets	30 seconds rest between sets

HINTS

• Keep your back upright by contracting your core muscles. Do not round your lower back. • Go through the full range of motion, from arms fully extended to dumbbells at shoulder level and back again.

#8 TWISTING CRUNCH

- Lie on your back on the ball in a reverse bridge position, with the ball in the middle of your back.

- Keep your head and neck off the ball and your feet flat on the ground.

- Place your hands to the sides of your head.

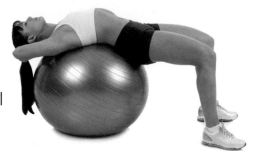

- Lift your head and shoulders up and away from the ball, and rotate them to one side by contracting your abdominals and twisting through the midsection.

- Twist back to the center, and roll your upper body back over the ball, returning to the starting position.

- Repeat in the opposite direction.

STRENGTH INTENSITY	TONE INTENSITY
3 sets	2 sets
15 reps	20 reps
45 seconds rest between sets	30 seconds rest between sets

HINTS

- Make sure to control the movement through your midsection, and avoid jerky motions. • You should not use your hands to pull your head and neck up. • Lift only your head and shoulders up off the ball, not your whole back.

#9 SIDE ROTATIONS

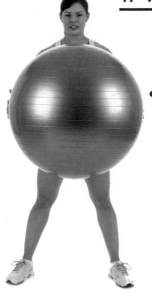

- Stand upright, holding the ball at waist height.

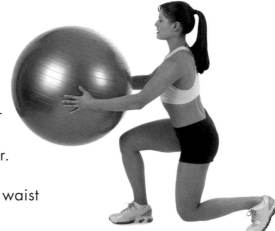

- Rotate to one side, bending your hips and knees and lowering your body down toward the floor.

- Switch sides, holding the ball at waist height throughout.

STRENGTH INTENSITY	TONE INTENSITY
3 sets	2 sets
15 reps	20 reps
45 seconds rest between sets	30 seconds rest between sets

HINTS

• Move through your hips and shoulders while also shifting your feet. • Keep your head up and look straight ahead to maintain a neutral spine.

#10 ELBOW BRIDGE

- Start with your forearms on the ball and your legs extended, with your feet on the floor.

- The ball should be directly under your chest, and your body should be straight.

- Hold this position for 10 seconds, and then lower your body down to lie on the ball.

- Repeat for the desired number of repetitions.

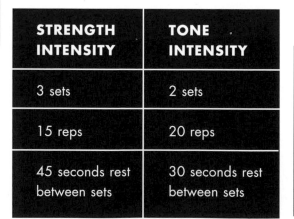

STRENGTH INTENSITY	TONE INTENSITY
3 sets	2 sets
15 reps	20 reps
45 seconds rest between sets	30 seconds rest between sets

HINTS

• To get into position, start in a kneeling position, with your elbows on the ball. Raise your hips up and hold your torso in this position throughout the movement.

• Make sure to keep your forearms on top of the ball.

#1 SIDE LUNGE

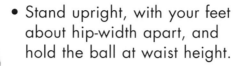

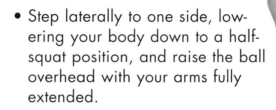

- Stand upright, with your feet about hip-width apart, and hold the ball at waist height.

- Step laterally to one side, lowering your body down to a half-squat position, and raise the ball overhead with your arms fully extended.

- Push off the outside foot to return to the starting position, and lower the ball back to waist height.

- Repeat the exercise on the other leg.

STRENGTH INTENSITY	TONE INTENSITY
3 sets	2 sets
15 reps	20 reps
45 seconds rest between sets	30 seconds rest between sets

HINTS

• In squatting exercises, the back position is very important. Always maintain a neutral position, and do not round your lower back. • Keep your head up, looking straight forward, and your shoulders back. • Place your weight over the leg you step out onto, and push off this leg to return to the middle. Keep the other leg straight throughout.

#2 RECIPROCAL PRESS

- Lie on your back on the ball in a reverse bridge position, with the ball between your shoulder blades.

- Keep your hips level with your shoulders, and your feet flat on the floor.

- Hold a dumbbell in each hand, with one at shoulder level and the other with the arm fully extended.

- Press the lower dumbbell up to a straight-arm position directly over your upper chest as you lower the extended-arm dumbbell down to shoulder level in a reciprocal motion.

- Lower the dumbbell by bending at the elbow and returning to shoulder level as you press the other dumbbell back up to the straight-arm position, to return to your starting position.

STRENGTH INTENSITY	TONE INTENSITY
3 sets	2 sets
15 reps	20 reps
45 seconds rest between sets	30 seconds rest between sets

HINTS

- Keep your hips in line with your shoulders. Do not let them sag or dip.
- Both dumbbells should be moving at the same time in a smooth reciprocal motion. • Keep the dumbbell directly over your chest. Do not let it move outward or inward.

#3 UNI CLOSE ROW

- Lie facedown with the ball under your mid-abdomen and your legs stretched out behind you.

- Hold a dumbbell in one hand with your arm extended to the side of the ball and your elbow slightly bent and the palm facing in. Place the other hand behind your back.

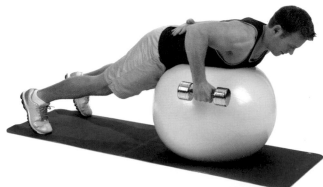

- Raise the dumbbell up by drawing your shoulder blade to the center of your back and bending your elbow.

- Lower the dumbbell back toward the floor to the starting position, extending at the elbow.

- Repeat on the other arm.

STRENGTH INTENSITY	TONE INTENSITY
3 sets	2 sets
15 reps	20 reps
45 seconds rest between sets	30 seconds rest between sets

HINTS

• Start with your feet about shoulder-width apart. • Draw your elbow up by your side, not outward. • Look down at the floor to keep your head in line with your spine.

#4 LEG EXTENSION

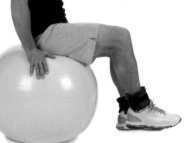

- Sit upright on the ball, with an ankle weight on each ankle and your feet flat on the floor.

- Place your hands to your sides on the ball.

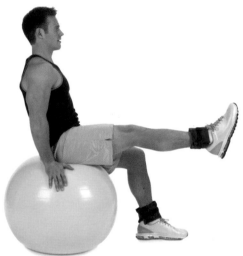

HINTS

- Keep one foot on the floor throughout the movement to maintain stability.
- Look straight ahead to keep your head and upper body level.

STRENGTH INTENSITY	TONE INTENSITY
3 sets	2 sets
15 reps	20 reps
45 seconds rest between sets	30 seconds rest between sets

- Lift one foot off the floor, and extend your leg straight out in front.

- Lower your leg, bending at the knee, and return to the starting position with both feet on the floor.

- Repeat the exercise on the other leg.

#5 FRONT RAISE

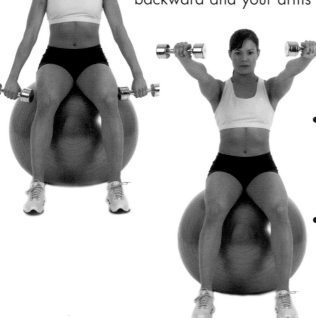

- Sit upright on the ball, with your feet flat on the floor.

- Hold a dumbbell in each hand with your palms facing backward and your arms extended by your sides.

- Raise the dumbbells up in front to just above shoulder level, keeping your arms straight.

- Lower the dumbbells back down to your sides, returning to the starting position with your arms fully extended.

STRENGTH INTENSITY	TONE INTENSITY
3 sets	2 sets
15 reps	20 reps
45 seconds rest between sets	30 seconds rest between sets

HINTS

- Contract your core muscles to keep your back upright as you raise the dumbbells up the sides. • Avoid jerky movements. • You can bend the elbows slightly to avoid too much stress on the shoulder joint.

#6 UNI HAMMER CURL

- Sit upright on the ball, with your feet flat on the floor.

- Hold a dumbbell in one hand, with your palm facing in and your arm extended by your side.

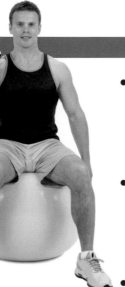

- Raise the dumbbell up in front to shoulder level, bending at the elbow, with your palm facing in.

- Lower the dumbbell by straightening your elbow and returning to the starting position, with your arm fully extended. Keep the other arm by your side throughout the movement.

- Repeat on the other side.

STRENGTH INTENSITY	TONE INTENSITY
3 sets	2 sets
15 reps	20 reps
45 seconds rest between sets	30 seconds rest between sets

HINTS

• Keep your back upright by contracting your core muscles. Do not round your lower back. • Go through the full range of motion, from arms fully extended to dumbbells at shoulder level and back again.

#7 DIP

- With the ball behind you, place your hands on top of the ball, with your arms straight and feet flat on the floor in front, knees slightly bent.

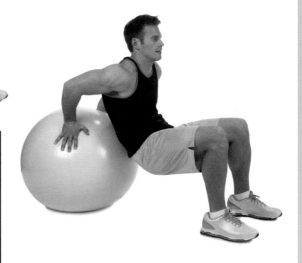

HINTS

- You can place the ball against a wall to prevent it from moving around.
- Do not sit on the ball in the down position; allow your lower back to barely touch the ball. • Keep your head up, and look straight forward.

- Lower your body toward the floor by bending at the elbows and going down till your lower back touches the ball.

- Push up against the ball to the starting position, where your arms are straight again.

- Keep your feet flat on the floor throughout the movement.

STRENGTH INTENSITY	TONE INTENSITY
3 sets	2 sets
15 reps	20 reps
45 seconds rest between sets	30 seconds rest between sets

#8 WEIGHTED CRUNCH

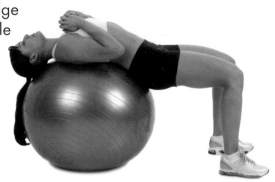

- Lie on your back in a reverse bridge position, with the ball in the middle of your back.

- Hold a dumbbell in both hands under your chin and close to your chest.

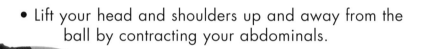

- Lift your head and shoulders up and away from the ball by contracting your abdominals.

- Roll your upper body back over the ball, returning to the starting position and keeping the dumbbell in the same position throughout.

STRENGTH INTENSITY	TONE INTENSITY
3 sets	2 sets
15 reps	20 reps
45 seconds rest between sets	30 seconds rest between sets

HINTS

- Make sure to control the movement through your midsection, and avoid jerky motions. • Keep the weight close to your chest, holding it in your hands.
- Lift only your head and shoulders up off the ball, not your whole back.

- Lie on one side, with your forearm on the ball and your legs stretched out. Place your other arm on your side.

- Hold this position for 10 seconds; then lower your hips back down to the ball.

- Repeat for the desired number of repetitions, and switch sides.

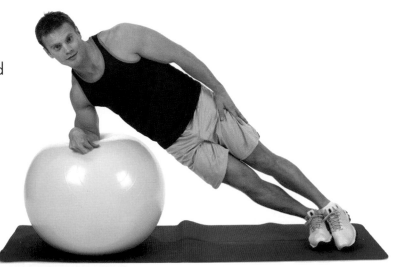

STRENGTH INTENSITY	TONE INTENSITY
3 sets	2 sets
15 reps	20 reps
45 seconds rest between sets	30 seconds rest between sets

HINTS

• Keep your upper body aligned with your hips; do not let your hips sag or dip and do not allow your shoulders to fall forward. • Look straight ahead to maintain a neutral spine.

#10 BRIDGE

- Lie on your back on the mat, with your heels on top of the ball.

- Place your hands on the mat by your sides.

- Raise your hips off the mat by contracting your core and abdominal muscles.

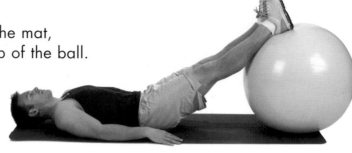

- Hold at the top for 10 seconds; then lower your body back to the mat, returning to the starting position.

- Repeat this movement, holding at the top for the desired number of repetitions.

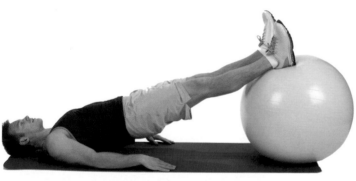

STRENGTH INTENSITY	TONE INTENSITY
3 sets	2 sets
15 reps	20 reps
45 seconds rest between sets	30 seconds rest between sets

HINTS

- Push your hands into the floor to help stabilize yourself when raising your hips. • Only your head, upper back, hands, and shoulders should be in contact with the mat at the top position.

#1 STEP UP

- Start with your arms fully extended overhead and with the ball in your hands.

- Place one foot up on a chair, and keep the other one flat on the floor.

- Lean forward, placing your body weight on the foot that is on the chair.

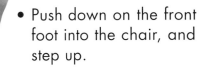

- Push down on the front foot into the chair, and step up.

- Keep the ball overhead with your arms fully extended throughout the movement.

STRENGTH INTENSITY	TONE INTENSITY
3 sets	2 sets
12 reps	15 reps
45 seconds rest between sets	30 seconds rest between sets

HINTS

- Keep your head up and look straight forward to maintain a neutral spine.
- Place your body weight on the foot that is on the chair, not on the back foot. Try not to push off using the back foot. Use the top foot to do the work.

#2 BENT-OVER ROW

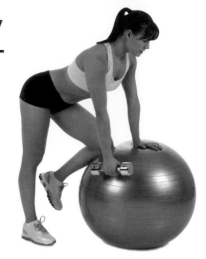

- Place one knee and the same-side hand on the ball.

- Hold a dumbbell in the other hand by your side, with your arm fully extended.

- Place the other foot flat on the floor a little behind and to the side of the ball.

- Raise the dumbbell up to your chest, bending at the elbow.

- Lower the dumbbell back to the starting position.

- Repeat on the other side.

STRENGTH INTENSITY	TONE INTENSITY
3 sets	2 sets
12 reps	15 reps
45 seconds rest between sets	30 seconds rest between sets

HINTS

• Look down toward the floor to maintain a neutral spine. • Do not lift your head as you lift the dumbbell. • Raise the dumbbell so your elbow comes above your shoulder.

#3 RECIPROCAL INCLINE PRESS

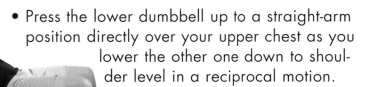

- Lie on your back on the ball in a reverse bridge position, with the ball between your shoulder blades.

- Drop your hips so your back lies on the ball, your body is at a 45-degree angle, and your feet are flat on the floor.

- Hold a dumbbell in each hand, with one at shoulder level and the other with the arm fully extended.

- Press the lower dumbbell up to a straight-arm position directly over your upper chest as you lower the other one down to shoulder level in a reciprocal motion.

- Lower the dumbbell by bending at the elbow and returning to shoulder level as you press the other dumbbell back up to the straight-arm position.

STRENGTH INTENSITY	TONE INTENSITY
3 sets	2 sets
12 reps	15 reps
45 seconds rest between sets	30 seconds rest between sets

HINTS

- Both dumbbells should be moving at the same time in a smooth reciprocal motion. • Keep the dumbbell directly over your chest; do not let it move outward or inward.

#4 LEG CURL

- Using ankle weights, start by lying facedown with the ball under your upper legs.

- Place your hands on the mat directly under your shoulders, with your arms fully extended.

- Your body should be in a straight line from head to feet.

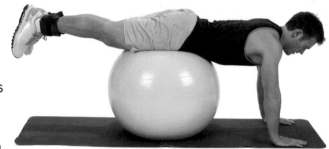

- Bring both feet to your buttocks, bending at the knees.

- Extend your legs, lowering your feet back to the starting position.

STRENGTH INTENSITY	TONE INTENSITY
3 sets	2 sets
12 reps	15 reps
45 seconds rest between sets	30 seconds rest between sets

HINTS

• To maintain a neutral spine, look at the floor and do not raise your head during the exercise. • Keep your arms fully extended throughout the movement. • Bring your feet all the way in to touch the buttocks and all the way back out to a straight-leg position.

#5 RECIPROCAL OVERHEAD PRESS

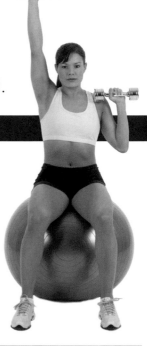

- Sit upright on the ball with your feet flat on the floor.

- Hold a dumbbell in each hand, with one at shoulder level and the other with the arm fully extended overhead.

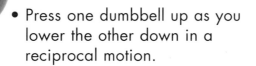

- Press one dumbbell up as you lower the other down in a reciprocal motion.

- Lower the dumbbell by bending at the elbow and returning to shoulder level as you press the other dumbbell back up to the straight-arm position.

STRENGTH INTENSITY	TONE INTENSITY
3 sets	2 sets
12 reps	15 reps
45 seconds rest between sets	30 seconds rest between sets

HINTS

- Keep your back upright by contracting your core muscles as you push the dumbbells overhead. Do not round your upper back. • Go through the full range of motion, from shoulder level to arm fully extended overhead and back again. • Both dumbbells should be moving at the same time in a smooth reciprocal motion.

#6 DUMBBELL FRENCH PRESS

- Lie on your back on the ball in a reverse bridge position, with the ball between your shoulder blades.

- Keep your hips level with your shoulders and your feet flat on the floor.

- Hold a dumbbell in each hand, with your elbows flexed and the weight positioned at the sides of your head (near your ears).

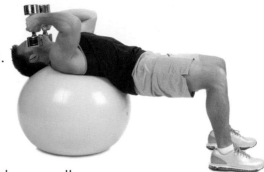

HINTS

- Keep your hips in line with your shoulders. Do not let them sag or dip. • Be careful not to bang the dumbbells against your head as you lift and lower them.
- Keep you shoulders steady; movement should occur only at the elbows.

STRENGTH INTENSITY	TONE INTENSITY
3 sets	2 sets
12 reps	15 reps
45 seconds rest between sets	30 seconds rest between sets

- Raise the dumbbells up until your arms are straight and the weights are overhead.

- Lower the dumbbells, bending at the elbows and returning to the starting position. Make sure to go all the way down till the dumbbells are back at the sides of your head.

#7 PREACHER CURL

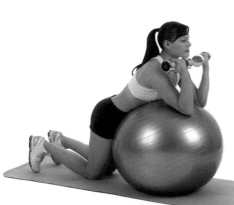

- Kneel on the mat with your chest and elbows on the ball, arms fully extended over the ball, and a dumbbell in each hand.

- Raise the dumbbells up in front to shoulder level, bending at the elbows, with your palms facing back.

- Lower the dumbbells by extending your elbows, returning to the starting position with your arms fully extended over the ball.

STRENGTH INTENSITY	TONE INTENSITY
3 sets	2 sets
12 reps	15 reps
45 seconds rest between sets	30 seconds rest between sets

HINTS

- Keep your shoulders and upper arms steady by pressing your elbows into the ball. • Be careful not to round your upper back as you curl up. Maintain a neutral spine throughout the movement.

#8 REVERSE CRUNCH

- Lie on your back on the mat, with the ball on the mat between your feet and with your knees bent.

- Place your hands at your sides.

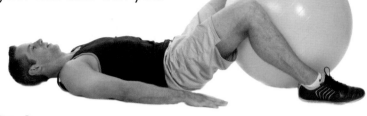

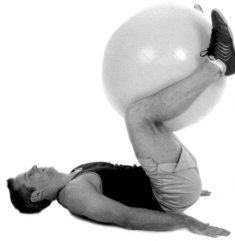

- Raise your hips and lower back off the mat, bringing your knees to your chest and the ball up.

- Return to starting position with your feet on the mat.

STRENGTH INTENSITY	TONE INTENSITY
3 sets	2 sets
12 reps	15 reps
45 seconds rest between sets	30 seconds rest between sets

HINTS

• Keep your upper back and shoulders on the mat. • Do not move your leg position. Keep your knees bent at the same angle throughout the movement.
• Make sure to go through the full range of motion, bringing the ball all the way down to the mat each time.

#9 UNI BRIDGE

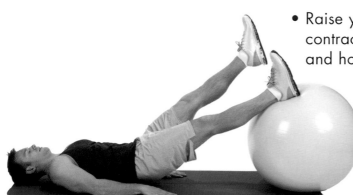

- Lie on your back on the mat, with your heels on the ball and your legs extended.

- Place your hands by your sides, and raise one foot off the ball.

- Raise your hips off the mat by contracting your abdominals, and hold this position.

- Lower your hips back to the mat, returning to the starting position and keeping one leg off the ball.

- Repeat on the other leg.

STRENGTH INTENSITY	TONE INTENSITY
3 sets	2 sets
12 reps	15 reps
45 seconds rest between sets	30 seconds rest between sets

HINTS

• Push your hands into the floor to help stabilize yourself when raising your hips. • Only your head, upper back, hands, and shoulders should be in contact with the mat at the top position.

#10 TORSO ROTATION

- Lie on your back in a reverse bridge position, with the ball between your shoulder blades and your feet flat on the floor. Keep your hips level with your shoulders.

- Hold one dumbbell in both hands, with your arms fully extended upward and the dumbbell directly over your chest.

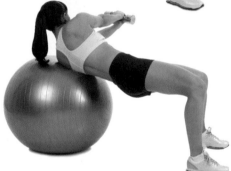

- Rotate your body to one side on the ball, rolling onto your shoulder and keeping your arms fully extended.

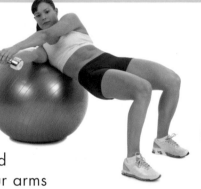

- Rotate back to the other side, going a full 180 degrees.

STRENGTH INTENSITY	TONE INTENSITY
3 sets	2 sets
12 reps	15 reps
45 seconds rest between sets	30 seconds rest between sets

HINTS

- Keep your hips in line with your shoulders. Do not let them sag or dip.
- This exercise requires you to contract the abdominal and core muscles.
- Rotate from side to side till the ball reaches shoulder level.

#1 UNI DEADLIFT

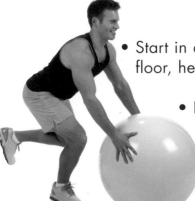

- Start in a squat position, with your feet flat on the floor, head up, and your back in a neutral position.

- Raise one foot off the floor, and hold the ball on the floor in front of you.

- Stand up and raise the ball overhead, with your arms fully extended, keeping one foot off the floor.

HINTS

- In squatting exercises, the back position is very important. Always maintain a neutral position, and do not round your lower back. • Keep your head up, looking straight forward, and your shoulders back to prevent rounding the upper back.

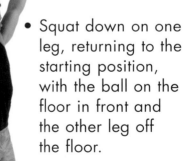

- Squat down on one leg, returning to the starting position, with the ball on the floor in front and the other leg off the floor.

- Repeat this exercise on the other leg.

STRENGTH INTENSITY	TONE INTENSITY
3 sets	2 sets
12 reps	15 reps
45 seconds rest between sets	30 seconds rest between sets

#2 PUSH-UP

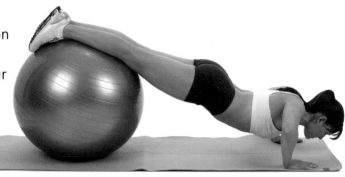

- Start with your hands on the mat directly under your shoulders and your feet on the ball.

- Your chest should be nearly touching the mat, and your body should be fully extended.

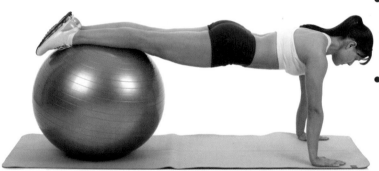

- Push up away from the mat, extending your arms fully.

- Lower your body back down to the mat again till your chest is nearly touching the mat.

STRENGTH INTENSITY	TONE INTENSITY
3 sets	2 sets
12 reps	15 reps
45 seconds rest between sets	30 seconds rest between sets

HINTS

• Start by lying on your stomach on the ball and walking your hands out while rolling the ball down your legs to your feet. • Make sure to go all the way down till your chest is nearly touching the mat and back up, extending your arms fully. • Look down at the floor to maintain a neutral spine.

#3 ROLL OUT

- Kneel on the mat with your forearms on the ball, elbows bent, and your chest nearly touching the ball.

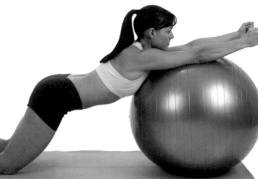

- Push the ball forward, extending your arms and keeping your upper body rigid.

- Pull the ball back, drawing your elbows in until you reach the starting position.

STRENGTH INTENSITY	TONE INTENSITY
3 sets	2 sets
12 reps	15 reps
45 seconds rest between sets	30 seconds rest between sets

HINTS

- Maintain a neutral spine by looking down and not moving your head.
- Control the movement through your midsection by keeping your abdominal and core muscles contracted, and avoid jerky motions.

#4 HIP ABDUCTION

- Lie on the mat on your side, with your legs extended and the ball between your feet.

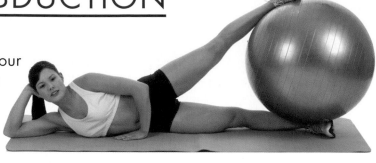

- Lift your legs and the ball up off the mat.

- Lower your legs and the ball, returning to the starting position with your leg on the mat.

- Repeat the exercise on the other side.

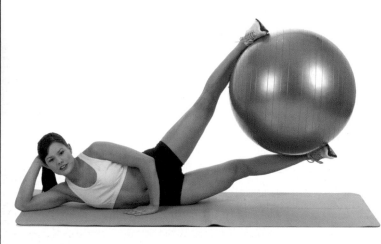

STRENGTH INTENSITY	TONE INTENSITY
3 sets	2 sets
12 reps	15 reps
45 seconds rest between sets	30 seconds rest between sets

HINTS

- Use your arms to support yourself as you complete the exercise. • Try to lift the ball as high as possible at the top of the movement. • Make sure to keep your upper body and shoulders in line with your hips, so that you do not fall forward.

#5 UNI OVERHEAD PRESS

- Sit upright on the ball, with your feet flat on the floor.

- Hold a dumbbell in one hand at shoulder level. Keep the other hand by your side.

- Push the dumbbell overhead, extending the arm.

- Lower the dumbbell by bending your elbow and returning to the starting position.

- Repeat this exercise on the other side.

STRENGTH INTENSITY	TONE INTENSITY
3 sets	2 sets
12 reps	15 reps
45 seconds rest between sets	30 seconds rest between sets

HINTS

• Keep your back upright by contracting your core muscles as you push the dumbbells overhead. Do not round your lower back. • Go through the full range of motion, from shoulder level to arm fully extended overhead and back again.

#6 UNI CURL

- Sit upright on the ball, holding a dumbbell with your arm extended by your side and with your palm out.

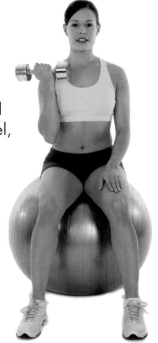

- Keep your other arm by your side.

- Raise the dumbbell up to shoulder level, finishing with your palm facing back. Do not turn your wrist as you raise the dumbbell.

- Repeat on the other arm.

STRENGTH INTENSITY	TONE INTENSITY
3 sets	2 sets
12 reps	15 reps
45 seconds rest between sets	30 seconds rest between sets

HINTS

- Keep your back upright by contracting your core muscles. Do not round your lower back. • Go through the full range of motion, from the arm fully extended to the dumbbell at shoulder level and back again.

• With the ball behind you, place your hands on top of the ball with your arms straight and feet flat on the floor in front, knees slightly bent.

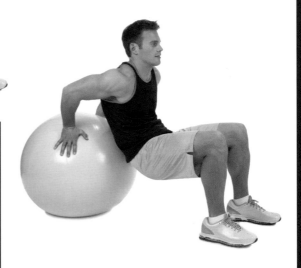

HINTS

• Do not sit on the ball in the down position; allow your lower back to barely touch the ball. • To increase the difficulty, you can straighten your legs and place your heels on the floor.
• Keep your head up and look straight forward throughout.

STRENGTH INTENSITY	TONE INTENSITY
3 sets	2 sets
12 reps	15 reps
45 seconds rest between sets	30 seconds rest between sets

• Lower your body toward the floor by bending at the elbows and going down till your lower back touches the ball.

• Push up against the ball to the starting position, where your arms are straight again.

• Keep your feet flat on the floor throughout the movement.

#8 LEG RAISE

- Lie on your back on the mat, with your legs straight and the ball between your feet.

- Place your hands by your sides.

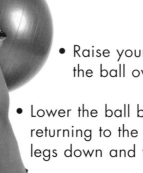

- Raise your legs up straight, bringing the ball over your midsection.

- Lower the ball by extending your hips, returning to the starting position with your legs down and the ball on the mat.

STRENGTH INTENSITY	TONE INTENSITY
3 sets	2 sets
12 reps	15 reps
45 seconds rest between sets	30 seconds rest between sets

HINTS

• Keep your head, back, and shoulders on the mat and keep your legs straight throughout the movement. • Push your hands into the floor to help stabilize yourself when raising your legs.

#9 TWISTING CRUNCH

- Lie on your back on the ball in a reverse bridge position with the ball in the middle of your back.

- Keep your head and neck off the ball and your feet flat on the ground.

- Place your hands to the sides of your head.

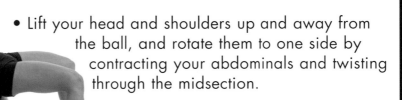

- Lift your head and shoulders up and away from the ball, and rotate them to one side by contracting your abdominals and twisting through the midsection.

- Twist back to the center, and roll your upper body back over the ball, returning to the starting position.

- Repeat in the other direction.

STRENGTH INTENSITY	TONE INTENSITY
3 sets	2 sets
12 reps	15 reps
45 seconds rest between sets	30 seconds rest between sets

HINTS

- Make sure to control the movement through your midsection, and avoid jerky motions. • You should not use your hands to pull your head and neck up. • Lift only your head and shoulders up off the ball, not your whole back.

#10 OBLIQUE CRUNCH

- Lie on one side on the ball, with both legs extended out and your feet on the mat.

- Place your hands to the sides of your head.

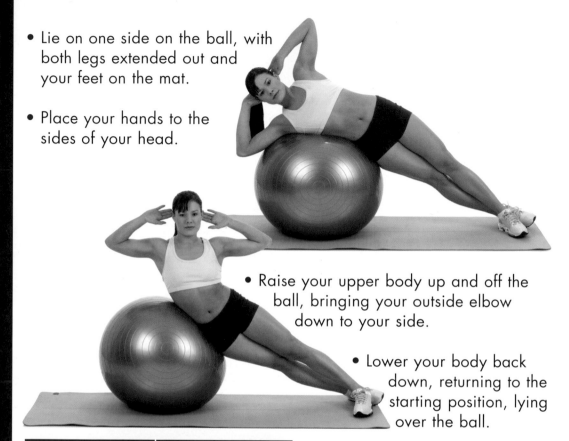

- Raise your upper body up and off the ball, bringing your outside elbow down to your side.

- Lower your body back down, returning to the starting position, lying over the ball.

STRENGTH INTENSITY	TONE INTENSITY
3 sets	2 sets
12 reps	15 reps
45 seconds rest between sets	30 seconds rest between sets

HINTS

- Make sure to control the movement through your midsection, and avoid jerky motions. • Keep your upper body upright, and do not allow your shoulders to fall forward or your elbows to come together.

#1 SQUAT TO BALL

- Start with the ball on the floor a little behind you.

- Standing upright with a dumbbell in each hand, place your feet facing forward about hip-width apart.

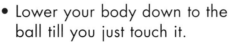

- Lower your body down to the ball till you just touch it.

- Keep your back in a neutral position.

- Push through the feet to return to the starting position.

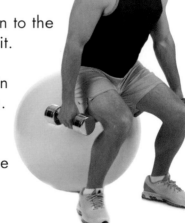

STRENGTH INTENSITY	TONE INTENSITY
3 sets	2 sets
12 reps	15 reps
45 seconds rest between sets	30 seconds rest between sets

HINTS

- In squatting exercises, the back position is very important. Maintain a neutral position, and do not round your lower back. • Keep your head up, looking straight forward, and your shoulders back.

#2 RECIPROCAL PRESS

- Lie on your back on the ball in a reverse bridge position, with the ball between your shoulder blades. Keep your hips level with your shoulders and your feet flat on the floor.

- Hold a dumbbell in each hand, with one at shoulder level and the other with the arm fully extended.

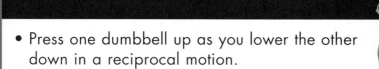

- Press one dumbbell up as you lower the other down in a reciprocal motion.

- Lower the dumbbell by bending at the elbow and returning to shoulder level as you press the other dumbbell back up to the straight-arm position, to return to your starting position.

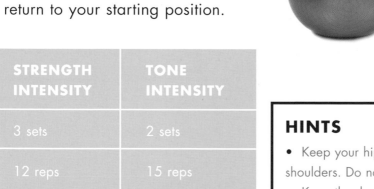

STRENGTH INTENSITY	TONE INTENSITY
3 sets	2 sets
12 reps	15 reps
45 seconds rest between sets	30 seconds rest between sets

HINTS

- Keep your hips in line with your shoulders. Do not let them sag or dip.
- Keep the dumbbell directly over your chest. Do not let it move outward or inward.

#3 RECIPROCAL WIDE ROW

- Lie facedown with the ball under your mid-abdomen and your legs stretched out behind.

- Hold a dumbbell in each hand, one at shoulder level and the other with your arm extended toward the floor.

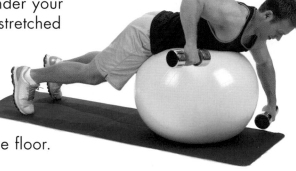

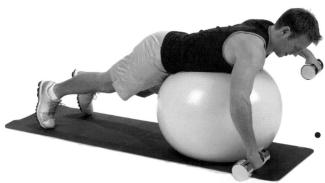

- Raise one dumbbell up, drawing your shoulder blade in and bending your elbow outward while at the same time lowering the other dumbbell to the floor in a reciprocal motion.

- Alternate the movement, making sure to go all the way down till one dumbbell is nearly at the floor and the other is at shoulder level.

STRENGTH INTENSITY	TONE INTENSITY
3 sets	2 sets
12 reps	15 reps
45 seconds rest between sets	30 seconds rest between sets

HINTS

- Start with your feet about shoulder-width apart. • Draw your elbows up and out to your sides, not in close.
- Look down at the floor to keep your head in line with your spine.

#4 BALL LEG CURL

- Lie on your back on the mat, with your heels on the ball and legs extended. Place your hands by your sides.

- Raise your hips off the mat by contracting your abdominals, and hold this position.

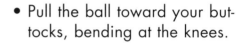

- Pull the ball toward your buttocks, bending at the knees.

- The ball should roll from your heels to the bottom of your feet.

- Extend your legs, returning the ball to the starting position, with your heels back on the ball.

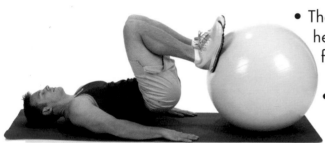

STRENGTH INTENSITY	TONE INTENSITY
3 sets	2 sets
12 reps	15 reps
45 seconds rest between sets	30 seconds rest between sets

HINTS

• Keep your core and abdominal muscles contracted, and maintain a neutral spine throughout the movement. • Push your hands into the floor to help stabilize yourself when drawing your knees in. • Only your head, upper back, hands, and shoulders should be in contact with the mat at the top position.

#5 DUMBBELL UNI FRENCH PRESS

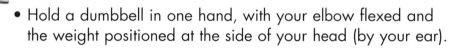

- Lie on your back on the ball in a reverse bridge position, with the ball between your shoulder blades.

- Keep your hips level with your shoulders and your feet flat on the floor.

- Hold a dumbbell in one hand, with your elbow flexed and the weight positioned at the side of your head (by your ear).

- Raise the dumbbell up until your arm is straight and the weight is overhead.

- Lower the dumbbell, bending at the elbow and returning to the starting position. Make sure to go all the way down till the dumbbell is back at the side of your head.

- Repeat on the opposite arm.

LEVEL 2: WORKOUT 3

STRENGTH INTENSITY	TONE INTENSITY
3 sets	2 sets
12 reps	15 reps
45 seconds rest between sets	30 seconds rest between sets

HINTS
- Keep your hips in line with your shoulders. Do not let them sag or dip.
- Be careful not to bang the dumbbell against your head as you lift and lower it. • Keep the shoulder steady; movement should occur only at the elbow.

#6 LATERAL RAISE

- Sit upright on the ball with your feet flat on the floor.

- Hold a dumbbell in each hand, with your palms facing in and your arms extended by your sides.

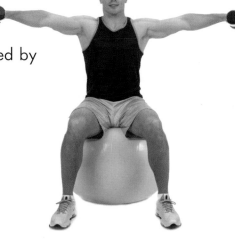

HINTS

- Keep your back upright by contracting your core muscles as you raise the dumbbells up the sides. • Avoid jerky movements.
- You can bend the elbows slightly to avoid too much stress on the shoulder joints.

- Raise the dumbbells up and out to the sides, going to just above shoulder level and keeping your arms straight.

- Lower the dumbbells back down to your sides, returning to the starting position with your arms fully extended.

STRENGTH INTENSITY	TONE INTENSITY
3 sets	2 sets
12 reps	15 reps
45 seconds rest between sets	30 seconds rest between sets

#7 UNI TWISTING CURL

- Sit upright on the ball, with your feet flat on the floor.

- Hold a dumbbell in one hand with your palm facing in and your arm extended by your side.

- Raise the dumbbell up in front to shoulder level, bending at the elbow and twisting at the wrist to finish with your palm facing back.

- Return the dumbbell to the starting position at your side. Keep the other arm by your side throughout the movement.

- Complete your repetitions, and then repeat on the other side.

STRENGTH INTENSITY	TONE INTENSITY
3 sets	2 sets
12 reps	15 reps
45 seconds rest between sets	30 seconds rest between sets

HINTS

- Keep your back upright by contracting your core muscles. Do not round your lower back. • Go through the full range of motion, from the arm fully extended to dumbbell at shoulder level and back again.

#8 WEIGHTED CRUNCH

- Lie on your back in a reverse bridge position, with the ball in the middle of your back.

- Hold one dumbbell in both hands under your chin and close to your chest.

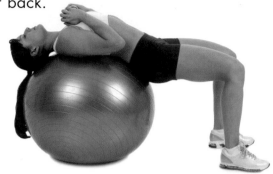

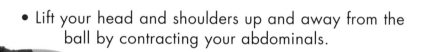

- Lift your head and shoulders up and away from the ball by contracting your abdominals.

- Roll your upper body back over the ball, returning to the starting position and keeping the dumbbell in the same position throughout.

STRENGTH INTENSITY	TONE INTENSITY
3 sets	2 sets
12 reps	15 reps
45 seconds rest between sets	30 seconds rest between sets

HINTS

• Make sure to control the movement through your midsection, and avoid jerky motions. • You should not use your hands to pull your head and neck up. • Lift only your head and shoulders up off the ball, not your whole back.

#9 TORSO ROTATION

- Lie on your back in a reverse bridge position, with the ball between your shoulder blades and your feet flat on the floor. Keep your hips level with your shoulders.

- Hold one dumbbell in both hands, with your arms fully extended upward and the dumbbell directly over your chest.

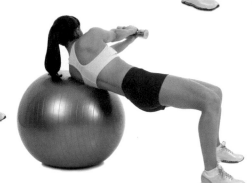

- Rotate your body to one side on the ball, rolling onto your shoulder and keeping your arms fully extended.

- Rotate back to the other side, going a full 180 degrees.

STRENGTH INTENSITY	TONE INTENSITY
3 sets	2 sets
12 reps	15 reps
45 seconds rest between sets	30 seconds rest between sets

HINTS

- Keep your hips in line with your shoulders. Do not let them sag or dip.
- This exercise requires you to contract the abdominal and core muscles.
- Rotate from side to side till the ball reaches shoulder level.

#10 KNEELING BACK EXTENSION

- Kneeling on the mat, lie with your chest on the ball and hands at the sides of your head.

- Let your head and shoulders drape over the ball.

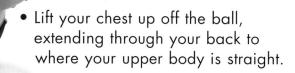

- Lift your chest up off the ball, extending through your back to where your upper body is straight.

- Keep your hands to the sides of your head, and return to the starting position with your chest on the ball.

STRENGTH INTENSITY	TONE INTENSITY
3 sets	2 sets
12 reps	15 reps
45 seconds rest between sets	30 seconds rest between sets

HINTS

- Lift only your head, shoulders, and chest up, not your whole upper body.
- Your upper body should be straight at the top of the movement. Do not overarch your lower back.

- Stand upright, holding the ball with your arms extended overhead.

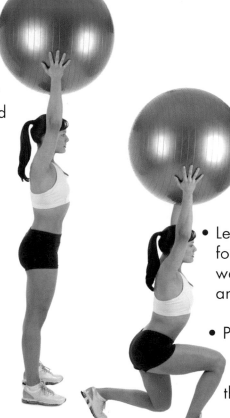

- Step forward, and drop your back knee down toward the floor, bending at the hip and knee.

- Lean your torso slightly forward, keeping all your weight on the front foot and the ball overhead.

- Push off the front foot to return to the starting position, and repeat on the other side.

STRENGTH INTENSITY	TONE INTENSITY
3 sets	2 sets
12 reps	15 reps
45 seconds rest between sets	30 seconds rest between sets

HINTS

- In squatting exercises, the back position is very important. Maintain a neutral position, and do not round your lower back. • Keep your head up, looking straight forward, and your shoulders back. • Place your weight over the leg you step out onto, and push off this leg to return to the middle.

#2 RECIPROCAL UPRIGHT ROW

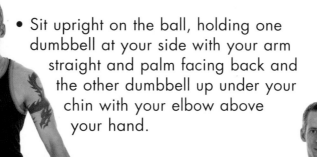

- Sit upright on the ball, holding one dumbbell at your side with your arm straight and palm facing back and the other dumbbell up under your chin with your elbow above your hand.

- Raise one dumbbell up under your chin while lowering the other dumbbell to your side. Both dumbbells should be moving at the same time but in opposite directions.

STRENGTH INTENSITY	TONE INTENSITY
3 sets	2 sets
12 reps	15 reps
45 seconds rest between sets	30 seconds rest between sets

HINTS

- When raising the dumbbells, make sure to bring your elbows higher than your shoulders at the top. • Do not turn your wrists. • Keep the dumbbells close to your body throughout.

#3 DUMBBELL PULLOVER

- Lie on your back in a reverse bridge position, with the ball between your shoulder blades and your feet flat on the floor. Keep your hips level with your shoulders.

- Hold one dumbbell in both hands, with your arms fully extended upward and the dumbbell directly over your chest.

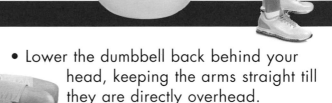

- Lower the dumbbell back behind your head, keeping the arms straight till they are directly overhead.

- Return the dumbbell to the starting position over your chest. Keep the arms completely straight throughout the movement.

STRENGTH INTENSITY	TONE INTENSITY
3 sets	2 sets
12 reps	15 reps
45 seconds rest between sets	30 seconds rest between sets

HINTS

- Keep your hips in line with your shoulders. Do not let them sag or dip.
- You can lower the dumbbell farther behind your head once you feel comfortable with the movement.

#4 UNI STIFF-LEG DEADLIFT

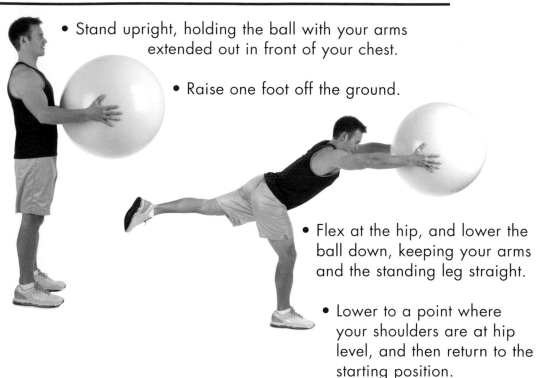

- Stand upright, holding the ball with your arms extended out in front of your chest.

- Raise one foot off the ground.

- Flex at the hip, and lower the ball down, keeping your arms and the standing leg straight.

- Lower to a point where your shoulders are at hip level, and then return to the starting position.

- Repeat the exercise, switching the legs.

STRENGTH INTENSITY	TONE INTENSITY
3 sets	2 sets
12 reps	15 reps
45 seconds rest between sets	30 seconds rest between sets

HINTS

- Keep your abdominal and core muscles activated during the movement. Do not round your lower back. • The standing leg should remain straight throughout the movement. A slight bend at the knee may help for people who have flexibility issues.

#5 REAR DELTOID ROW

- Lie facedown, with the ball under your mid-abdomen and your legs stretched out behind.

- Hold a dumbbell in each hand, with your elbows slightly bent and palms facing each other.

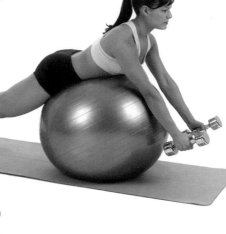

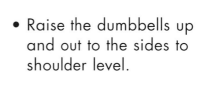

- Raise the dumbbells up and out to the sides to shoulder level.

- Keep your arms straight throughout the movement, and do not round the upper back.

STRENGTH INTENSITY	TONE INTENSITY
3 sets	2 sets
12 reps	15 reps
45 seconds rest between sets	30 seconds rest between sets

HINTS

- Start with your feet about shoulder-width apart. • Draw your arms up and out to the sides, pulling your shoulder blades together at the top. • Look down at the floor to keep your head in line with your spine.

#6 UNI PREACHER CURL

- Kneel on the mat, with your chest and elbows on the ball, arms fully extended over the ball, and a dumbbell in one hand. Keep the other hand down to the side of the ball.

HINTS

- Keep your shoulders and upper arms steady by pressing your elbow into the ball. • Be careful not to round your upper back as you curl up. Maintain a neutral spine throughout the movement.

- Raise the dumbbell up in front to shoulder level, bending at the elbow, with your palm facing back.

- Lower the dumbbell by extending your elbow, returning to the starting position with your arm fully extended over the ball.

- Complete your repetitions, and then switch to the other side.

STRENGTH INTENSITY	TONE INTENSITY
3 sets	2 sets
12 reps	15 reps
45 seconds rest between sets	30 seconds rest between sets

#7 CHAIR DIP

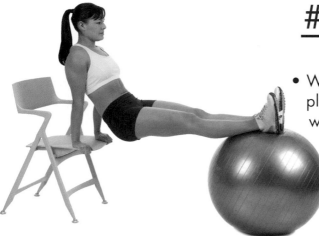

- With the ball in front of you, place your hands on a chair with your arms straight and your feet on the ball with your legs straight.

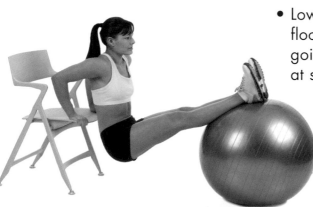

- Lower your body toward the floor by bending at the elbows, going down till your elbows are at shoulder level.

  - Push up against the chair to the starting position, where your arms are straight again.

STRENGTH INTENSITY	TONE INTENSITY
3 sets	2 sets
12 reps	15 reps
45 seconds rest between sets	30 seconds rest between sets

HINTS

- Start by sitting on the chair with your feet on the ball. Slowly push the ball out with your feet, and position your hands on the edge of the chair. • You can go lower than elbows to shoulder level once you feel comfortable with the movement.

#8 SIDE BRIDGE

- Lie on one side, with your forearm on the ball and your legs stretched out. Place your other arm on your side.

- Lift your hips off the ball and hold this position for 10 seconds; then lower your hips back down to the ball.

- Repeat for the desired number of repetitions, and switch sides.

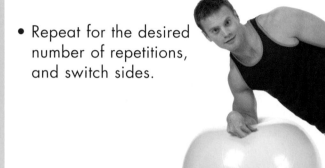

STRENGTH INTENSITY	TONE INTENSITY
3 sets	2 sets
12 reps	15 reps
45 seconds rest between sets	30 seconds rest between sets

HINTS

• Keep your upper body aligned with your hips. Do not let your hips sag or dip and do not allow your shoulders to fall forward. • Look straight ahead to maintain a neutral spine.

#9 BALL CRUNCH

- Lie on your back on the ball in a reverse bridge position, with the ball in the middle of your back.

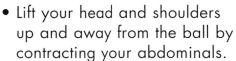

- Keep your head and neck off the ball and your feet flat on the ground.

- Place your hands to the sides of your head.

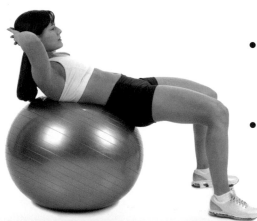

- Lift your head and shoulders up and away from the ball by contracting your abdominals.

- Roll your upper body back over the ball, returning to the starting position.

STRENGTH INTENSITY	TONE INTENSITY
3 sets	2 sets
12 reps	15 reps
45 seconds rest between sets	30 seconds rest between sets

HINTS

• Make sure to control the movement through your midsection, and avoid jerky motions. • You should not use your hands to pull your head and neck up. • Lift only your head and shoulders up off the ball, not your whole back.

#10 ALTERNATING FLYER

- Lie facedown, with the ball under your abdomen and both hands and feet touching the floor.

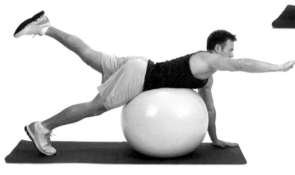

- Raise one arm and the opposite leg off the floor, keeping them straight.

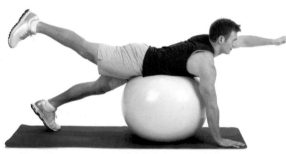

- Lower your arm and leg back to the starting position, and repeat with the other arm and opposite leg.

STRENGTH INTENSITY	TONE INTENSITY
3 sets	2 sets
12 reps	15 reps
45 seconds rest between sets	30 seconds rest between sets

HINTS
- Keep the ball under your abdomen to maintain balance. • Raise the arm and leg up in line with your hip and shoulder. • You should feel like you are stretching out and lengthening your spine.

#1 UNI SQUAT

- Start with ball on the floor behind you. Place your feet facing forward, hip-width apart. Raise one foot off floor.

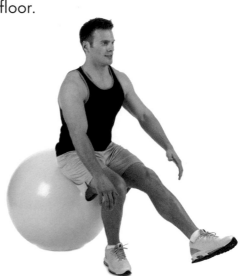

HINTS

- In squatting exercises, the back position is very important. Maintain a neutral position, and do not round your lower back.
- Keep your head up, looking straight forward, and your shoulders back.

STRENGTH INTENSITY	TONE INTENSITY
3 sets	2 sets
10 reps	15 reps
45 seconds rest between sets	30 seconds rest between sets

- Lower your body down to the ball till you just touch it, keeping one foot in the air with the leg out front. Keep your back in a neutral position.

- Push through the standing foot to return to the starting position.

#2 RECIPROCAL CLOSE ROW

- Lie facedown, with the ball under your mid-abdomen and your legs stretched out behind you.

- Hold a dumbbell in each hand, with palms facing in, one at shoulder level and the other with your arm extended toward the floor.

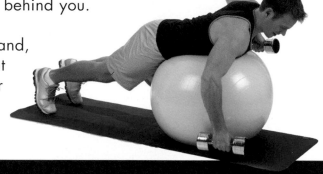

- Raise one dumbbell up, drawing your shoulder blade in and bending your elbow while at the same time lowering the other dumbbell to the floor in a reciprocal motion.

- Alternate the movement, making sure to go all the way down till one dumbbell is nearly at the floor and the other is nearly in the armpit.

STRENGTH INTENSITY	TONE INTENSITY
3 sets	2 sets
10 reps	15 reps
45 seconds rest between sets	30 seconds rest between sets

HINTS

• Start with your feet about shoulder-width apart. • Draw your elbows up by your sides, not outward. • Look down at the floor to keep your head in line with your spine.

#3 LEG EXTENSION

• Sit upright on the ball, with an ankle weight on each ankle and your feet flat on the floor. Place your hands on your hips.

• Lift one foot off the floor, and extend your leg straight out in front.

• Lower your leg, bending at the knee and returning to the starting position with both feet on the floor.

• Repeat the exercise on the other leg.

STRENGTH INTENSITY	TONE INTENSITY
3 sets	2 sets
10 reps	15 reps
45 seconds rest between sets	30 seconds rest between sets

HINTS

• Keep one foot on the floor throughout the movement to maintain stability.
• Keep your head and upper body level by placing your hands on your hips and looking straight ahead.

#4 DUMBBELL INCLINE PRESS

- Lie on your back on the ball in a reverse bridge position, with the ball between your shoulder blades.

- Drop your hips so your back lies on the ball and your body is at a 45-degree angle with your feet flat on the floor.

- Hold a dumbbell in each hand at shoulder level.

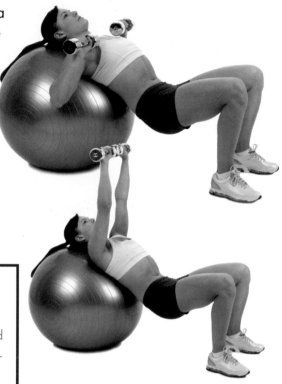

HINTS

- Although your back is on the ball, you must keep the abdominal muscles contracted to help keep you stable. • Keep the dumbbells directly over your chest. Do not let them move outward or inward.

STRENGTH INTENSITY	TONE INTENSITY
3 sets	2 sets
10 reps	15 reps
45 seconds rest between sets	30 seconds rest between sets

- Press the dumbbells up until your arms are straight and the dumbbells are directly over your upper chest.

- Lower the dumbbells by bending at the elbows and returning to the starting position. Make sure to go all the way down till the dumbbells are back to shoulder level.

#5 RECIPROCAL OVERHEAD PRESS

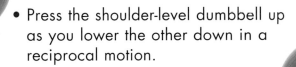

- Sit upright on the ball with your feet flat on the floor.

- Hold a dumbbell in each hand, with one at shoulder level and the other with the arm fully extended overhead.

- Press the shoulder-level dumbbell up as you lower the other down in a reciprocal motion.

- Lower the dumbbell by bending at the elbow and returning to shoulder level as you press the other dumbbell back up to the straight-arm position.

STRENGTH INTENSITY	TONE INTENSITY
3 sets	2 sets
10 reps	15 reps
45 seconds rest between sets	30 seconds rest between sets

HINTS

• Keep your back upright by contracting your core muscles as you push the dumbbells overhead. Do not round your lower back. • Go through the full range of motion, from shoulder level to arms fully extended overhead and back again. • Both dumbbells should be moving at the same time in a smooth reciprocal motion.

#6 UNI KNEELING EXTENSION

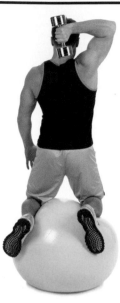

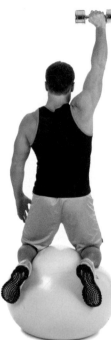

- Kneel upright on the ball.

- Hold a dumbbell in one hand behind your head with your elbow bent.

- Lift the dumbbell by extending your elbow and straightening your arm directly overhead.

- Lower the dumbbell to the starting position behind your head.

- Repeat on the other side.

STRENGTH INTENSITY	TONE INTENSITY
3 sets	2 sets
10 reps	15 reps
45 seconds rest between sets	30 seconds rest between sets

HINTS

- Practice kneeling on the ball before attempting the exercise with weights.
- Be careful not to bang the dumbbell against the back of your head as you lift and lower it. • Go through the full range of motion, from behind the head to the arm fully extended overhead and back again. • Keep your shoulder steady; movement should occur only at the elbow.

#7 RECIPROCAL HAMMER CURL

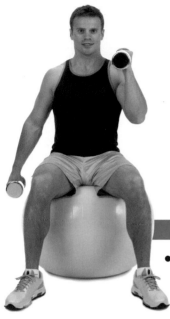

- Sit upright on the ball, with your feet flat on the floor.

- Hold a dumbbell in each hand with palms facing in.

- Start with one dumbbell at shoulder level and the other with the arm fully extended by your side.

- Raise the lower dumbbell up to shoulder level as you lower the other down to your side in a reciprocal motion.

- Return the dumbbells to the starting positions, where one dumbbell is back to shoulder level and the other is extended by your side.

STRENGTH INTENSITY	TONE INTENSITY
3 sets	2 sets
10 reps	15 reps
45 seconds rest between sets	30 seconds rest between sets

HINTS

• Keep your back upright by contracting your core muscles. • Go through the full range of motion, from arm fully extended to dumbbell at shoulder level and back again.

#8 FLAT FLY

- Lie on your back in a reverse bridge position, with the ball between your shoulder blades. Keep your hips level with your shoulders.

- Hold a dumbbell in each hand, with your arms fully extended overhead and your palms facing in. Keep a slight bend in the elbows throughout the movement.

HINT

- Keep your hips in line with your shoulders. Do not let them sag or dip.

STRENGTH INTENSITY	TONE INTENSITY
3 sets	2 sets
10 reps	15 reps
45 seconds rest between sets	30 seconds rest between sets

- Lower the dumbbells out to the sides and down to shoulder level.

- Return to the starting position, coming all the way back to a fully extended position overhead.

#9 UNI LATERAL RAISE

- Sit upright on the ball, with your feet flat on the floor.

- Hold a dumbbell in one hand, with your palm facing in and your arm extended by your side. Keep the other hand by your side or on your knee.

- Raise the dumbbell up and out to just above shoulder level, keeping this arm straight and the other arm by your side.

- Return the dumbbell to the starting position at your side.

- Repeat on the other side.

STRENGTH INTENSITY	TONE INTENSITY
3 sets	2 sets
10 reps	15 reps
45 seconds rest between sets	30 seconds rest between sets

HINTS

• Keep your back upright by contracting your core muscles as you raise the dumbbell up to the side. • Avoid jerky movements. • You can bend the elbow slightly to avoid too much stress on the shoulder joint.

#10 LEG RAISE

- Lie on your back on the mat, with your legs straight and the ball between your feet.

- Place your hands by your sides.

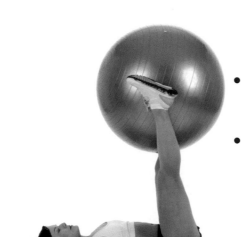

- Raise your legs up straight, bringing the ball over your midsection.

- Lower the ball by extending your hips, returning to the starting position with your legs down and the ball on the mat.

STRENGTH INTENSITY	TONE INTENSITY
3 sets	2 sets
10 reps	15 reps
45 seconds rest between sets	30 seconds rest between sets

HINTS

• Keep your head, back, and shoulders on the mat. • Keep your legs straight throughout the movement. • You can use your hands to help stabilize yourself and push into the floor when raising your hips.

#1 DUMBBELL FOOT-UP SPLIT SQUAT

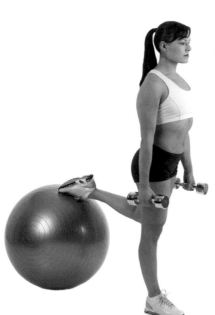

- Start with the ball on the floor behind you.

- Place one foot on top of the ball and the other foot out in front on the floor.

- Hold a dumbbell in each hand, and keep your weight on the leg out in front.

- Lower your body down till your back shin touches the ball.

- Keep your back in a neutral position and push through the front foot to return to the starting position.

STRENGTH INTENSITY	TONE INTENSITY
3 sets	2 sets
10 reps	15 reps
45 seconds rest between sets	30 seconds rest between sets

HINTS

• In squatting exercises, the back position is very important. Maintain a neutral position, and do not round your lower back. • Keep your head up, and look straight forward to maintain a neutral spine.

#2 WALK AROUND

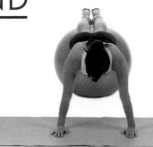

- Start with your hands on the mat directly under your shoulders, with your arms fully extended and your feet on the ball.

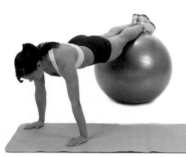

- Lift one hand, and move it to one side, following with the other hand.

- Continue moving your hands as you walk them from one side to the other.

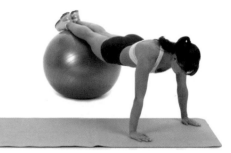

- Reverse the direction, and walk on your hands back to the starting position.

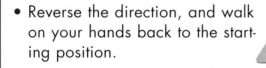

STRENGTH INTENSITY	TONE INTENSITY
3 sets	2 sets
10 reps	15 reps
45 seconds rest between sets	30 seconds rest between sets

HINTS

- Start by taking small steps with your hands. You can increase the distance of the steps once you are used to the movement. • Look down at the floor to maintain a neutral spine.

#3 UNI WIDE ROW

- Lie facedown with the ball under your mid-abdomen and your legs stretched out behind you.

- Hold a dumbbell in one hand, with your elbow slightly bent and facing out to the side. Place the other hand behind your back.

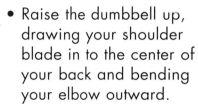

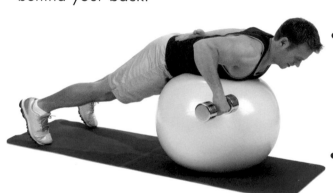

- Raise the dumbbell up, drawing your shoulder blade in to the center of your back and bending your elbow outward.

- Lower the dumbbell back toward the floor, extending at the elbow.

- Repeat this exercise on the other side.

STRENGTH INTENSITY	TONE INTENSITY
3 sets	2 sets
10 reps	15 reps
45 seconds rest between sets	30 seconds rest between sets

HINTS

- Start with your feet about shoulder-width apart. • Draw your elbows up and out to your sides, not in close.
- Look down at the floor to keep your head in line with your spine.

#4 BALL LEG CURL

- Lie on your back on the mat with your heels on the ball and legs extended. Place your hands by your sides.

- Raise your hips off the mat by contracting your abdominals, and hold this position.

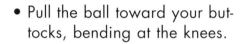

- Pull the ball toward your buttocks, bending at the knees.

- The ball should roll from your heels to the bottom of your feet.

- Extend your legs, returning the ball to the starting position, with your heels back on the ball.

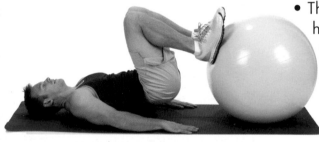

STRENGTH INTENSITY	TONE INTENSITY
3 sets	2 sets
10 reps	15 reps
45 seconds rest between sets	30 seconds rest between sets

HINTS
• Keep your core and abdominal muscles contracted, and maintain a neutral spine throughout the movement. • Push your hands into the floor to help stabilize yourself when drawing your knees in. • Only your head, upper back, hands, and shoulders should be in contact with the mat at the top position.

#5 WALL SQUAT TO PRESS

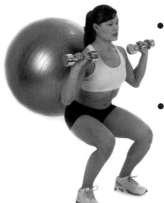

- Start with the ball against the wall and at lower-back level. Place your feet ahead of ball, hip-width apart. Hold a dumbbell in each hand.

- Lower your body down toward the floor, pushing slightly against the ball. Stop when your thighs are parallel to the floor.

- Holding this squat position, push the dumbbells overhead, extending the arms.

- Return the dumbbells to the starting position, making sure to go all the way down till the dumbbells are at shoulder level. Stand straight again.

STRENGTH INTENSITY	TONE INTENSITY
3 sets	2 sets
10 reps	15 reps
45 seconds rest between sets	30 seconds rest between sets

HINTS

- Keep your head up, and look straight ahead throughout the movement. Do not look down at the floor or at your feet. • Make sure to keep your feet flat on the floor, with your heel down, as you move up and down.
- Keep pushing back against the ball throughout the movement.

#6 RECIPROCAL CURL

- Sit upright on the ball, with your feet flat on the floor.

- Hold a dumbbell in each hand, starting with one at shoulder level and palm facing back and the other with the arm fully extended by your side and palm facing forward.

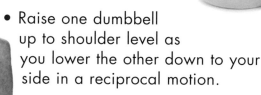

- Raise one dumbbell up to shoulder level as you lower the other down to your side in a reciprocal motion.

- Return the dumbbells to the starting positions, where one dumbbell is back to shoulder level and the other is extended by your side.

STRENGTH INTENSITY	TONE INTENSITY
3 sets	2 sets
10 reps	15 reps
45 seconds rest between sets	30 seconds rest between sets

HINTS

• Keep your back upright by contracting your core muscles. • Go through the full range of motion, from arm fully extended to dumbbell at shoulder level and back again.

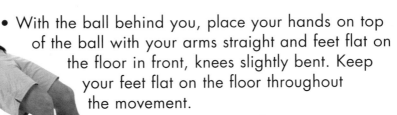

- With the ball behind you, place your hands on top of the ball with your arms straight and feet flat on the floor in front, knees slightly bent. Keep your feet flat on the floor throughout the movement.

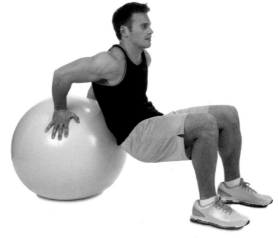

HINTS

- You can place the ball against a wall to prevent it from moving around.
- Do not sit on the ball in the down position; allow your lower back to barely touch the ball. • To increase the difficulty, you can straighten your legs and place your heels on the floor.

STRENGTH INTENSITY	TONE INTENSITY
3 sets	2 sets
10 reps	15 reps
45 seconds rest between sets	30 seconds rest between sets

- Lower your body toward the floor by bending at the elbows and going down till your lower back touches the ball.

- Push up against the ball to the starting position, where your arms are straight again.

#8 UNI FRONT RAISE

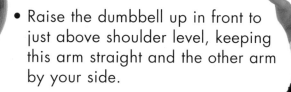

- Sit upright on the ball, with your feet flat on the floor.

- Hold a dumbbell in one hand, with your palm facing backward and your arm extended by your side. Keep the other hand by your side or on your knee.

- Raise the dumbbell up in front to just above shoulder level, keeping this arm straight and the other arm by your side.

- Return the dumbbell to the starting position at your side.

- Repeat to finish your reps, then switch to the other side.

STRENGTH INTENSITY	TONE INTENSITY
3 sets	2 sets
10 reps	15 reps
45 seconds rest between sets	30 seconds rest between sets

HINTS

- Keep your back upright by contracting your core muscles as you raise the dumbbell. • Avoid jerky movements.
- You can bend the elbow slightly to avoid too much stress on the shoulder joint.

LEVEL 3: WORKOUT 2

- Start with your hands on the mat directly under your shoulders, with your arms fully extended and your shins on the ball.

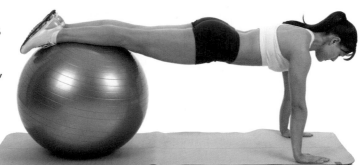

- Drag the ball toward your hands, bending your knees and bringing them to your chest.

- Extend your knees and straighten your legs, returning the ball to the starting position.

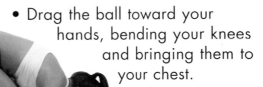

STRENGTH INTENSITY	TONE INTENSITY
3 sets	2 sets
10 reps	15 reps
45 seconds rest between sets	30 seconds rest between sets

HINTS

- Keep your hips in line with your shoulders. Do not let them sag or dip.
- Look down at the floor to maintain a neutral spin. • Make sure to keep your hands under your shoulders throughout the movement.

#10 BACK EXTENSTION

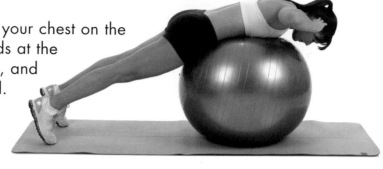

- Lie facedown with your chest on the ball and your hands at the sides of your head, and your legs extended.

- Let your head and shoulders drape over the ball.

- Lift your chest up off the ball, extending through your back.

- Keep your hands to the sides of your head, and return to the starting position with your chest on the ball.

STRENGTH INTENSITY	TONE INTENSITY
3 sets	2 sets
10 reps	15 reps
45 seconds rest between sets	30 seconds rest between sets

HINTS

- Lift only your head and shoulders up, not your whole upper body. • Your upper body should be straight at the top of the movement. • Push your toes into the floor to help keep you stable and maintain your grip.

#1 LUNGE

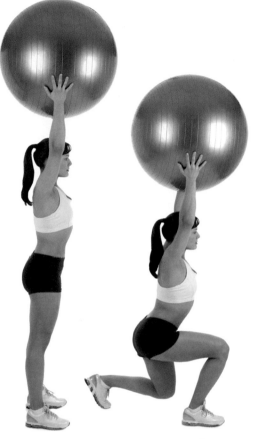

- Stand upright, holding the ball overhead with your arms extended.

- Step forward and drop your back knee down toward the floor, bending at the hip and knee.

- Lean your torso slightly forward, keeping all your weight on the front foot and the ball overhead.

- Push off the front foot to return to the starting position, and repeat on the other side.

STRENGTH INTENSITY	TONE INTENSITY
3 sets	2 sets
10 reps	15 reps
45 seconds rest between sets	30 seconds rest between sets

HINTS

• In squatting exercises, the back position is very important. Maintain a neutral position, and do not round your lower back. • Keep your head up, looking straight forward, and your shoulders back. • Place your weight over the leg you step out onto, and push off this leg to return to the middle. Keep the other leg straight throughout.

#2 PUSH-UP ON BALL

- Start with your hands on the ball directly under your shoulders and your legs extended with your feet on the floor.

- Your chest should be nearly touching the ball, and your body should be fully extended.

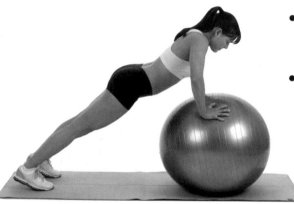

- Push up away from the ball, extending your arms fully.

- Lower your body back down to the ball, returning to the starting position, where your chest is again nearly touching the ball.

STRENGTH INTENSITY	TONE INTENSITY
3 sets	2 sets
10 reps	15 reps
45 seconds rest between sets	30 seconds rest between sets

HINTS

- Start in a kneeling position, with your hands on the ball. Raise your hips up, and hold your torso in this position throughout the movement. • Make sure to go all the way up, extending your arms fully, and all the way down till your chest is nearly touching the ball.

#3 ONE-LEG UNI CLOSE ROW

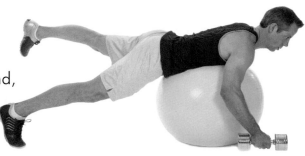

- Lie facedown with the ball under your mid-abdomen, your legs stretched out behind, and one foot slightly off the ground. Keep this foot off the ground throughout the movement.

- Hold a dumbbell in the opposite hand, with the elbow slightly bent.

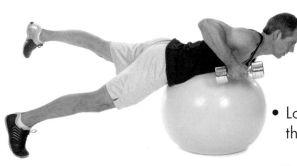

- Raise the dumbbell up, drawing your shoulder blade in and bending your elbow.

- Lower the dumbbell back toward the floor, extending at the elbow.

- Repeat this exercise on the other side.

STRENGTH INTENSITY	TONE INTENSITY
3 sets	2 sets
10 reps	15 reps
45 seconds rest between sets	30 seconds rest between sets

HINTS

• Draw your elbow up by your side, not outward. • Look down at the floor to keep your head in line with your spine. • Keep your leg about 12 inches off the floor throughout the movement.

#4 UNI STIFF-LEG DEADLIFT

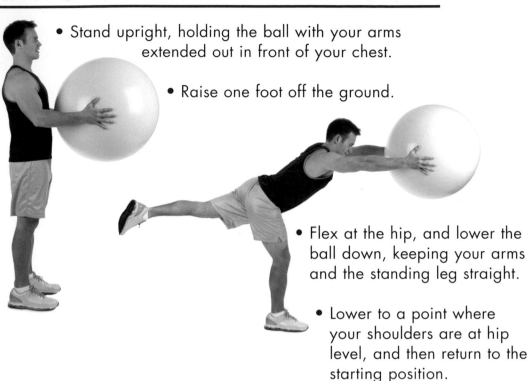

- Stand upright, holding the ball with your arms extended out in front of your chest.

- Raise one foot off the ground.

- Flex at the hip, and lower the ball down, keeping your arms and the standing leg straight.

- Lower to a point where your shoulders are at hip level, and then return to the starting position.

- Repeat the exercise, switching the legs.

STRENGTH INTENSITY	TONE INTENSITY
3 sets	2 sets
10 reps	15 reps
45 seconds rest between sets	30 seconds rest between sets

HINTS

- Keep your abdominal and core muscles activated during the movement. Do not round your lower back. • The standing leg should remain straight throughout the movement. • A slight bend at the knee may help people who have flexibility issues.

#5 KNEELING OVERHEAD PRESS

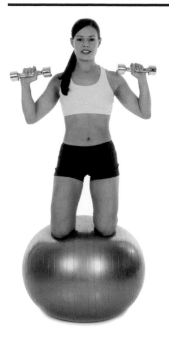

- Kneel upright on the ball, holding a dumbbell in each hand at shoulder level with your palms facing forward.

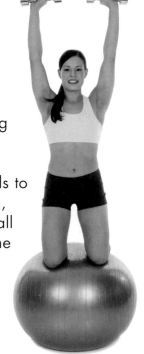

- Push the dumbbells overhead, extending the arms.

- Return the dumbbells to the starting position, making sure to go all the way down till the dumbbells are at shoulder level.

STRENGTH INTENSITY	TONE INTENSITY
3 sets	2 sets
10 reps	15 reps
45 seconds rest between sets	30 seconds rest between sets

HINTS

- Practice kneeling on the ball before attempting the exercise with weights.
- Go through the full range of motion, from shoulder level to arms fully extended overhead and back again.

#6 RECIPROCAL TWISTING CURL

- Sit upright on the ball, with your feet flat on the floor.

- Hold a dumbbell in each hand, starting with one at shoulder level and palm facing back and the other with the arm fully extended by your side and palm facing in.

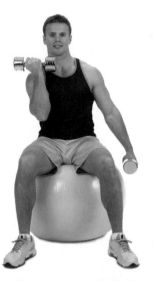

- Raise one dumbbell up to shoulder level as you lower the other down to your side in a reciprocal motion.

- Return the dumbbells to the starting positions, where one dumbbell is back to shoulder level and the other is extended by your side.

STRENGTH INTENSITY	TONE INTENSITY
3 sets	2 sets
10 reps	15 reps
45 seconds rest between sets	30 seconds rest between sets

HINTS

• Keep your back upright by contracting your core muscles. • Go through the full range of motion, from arm fully extended to dumbbell at shoulder level and back again.

#7 CHAIR DIP

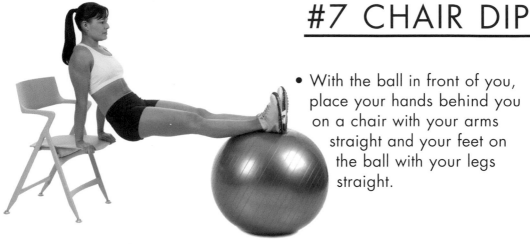

- With the ball in front of you, place your hands behind you on a chair with your arms straight and your feet on the ball with your legs straight.

- Lower your body toward the floor by bending at the elbows, going down till your elbows are at shoulder level.

- Push up against the chair to the starting position, where your arms are straight again.

STRENGTH INTENSITY	TONE INTENSITY
3 sets	2 sets
10 reps	15 reps
45 seconds rest between sets	30 seconds rest between sets

HINTS

- Start by sitting on the chair with your feet on the ball. Slowly push the ball out with your feet, and position your hands on the edge of the chair. • You can go lower than your elbows to shoulder level once you feel comfortable with the movement.

#8 HIP RAISE

- Lie on your back on the mat, with the ball between your feet and your legs straight up.

- Place your hands at your sides.

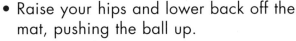

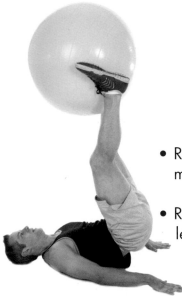

- Raise your hips and lower back off the mat, pushing the ball up.

- Return to the starting position, with your legs straight up.

STRENGTH INTENSITY	TONE INTENSITY
3 sets	2 sets
10 reps	15 reps
45 seconds rest between sets	30 seconds rest between sets

HINTS

• Keep your upper back and shoulders on the mat and keep your legs straight throughout the movement. • Push your hands into the floor to help stabilize yourself when raising your hips. • Only your head, upper back, hands, and shoulders should be in contact with the mat at the top position.

#9 WEIGHTED BACK EXTENSION

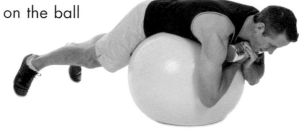

- Lie facedown with your chest on the ball and your legs extended.

- Hold a dumbbell in both hands under your chin, and let your head and shoulders drape over the ball.

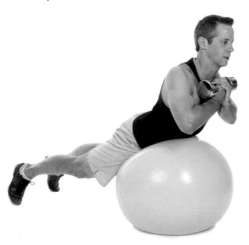

- Lift your chest up off the ball, extending through your back with the weight still under your chin.

- Lower your upper body by flexing at the midsection, returning to the starting position with your chest on the ball.

STRENGTH INTENSITY	TONE INTENSITY
3 sets	2 sets
10 reps	15 reps
45 seconds rest between sets	30 seconds rest between sets

HINTS

- Lift only your head, chest, and shoulders up, not your whole upper body.
- Your upper body should be straight at the top of the movement. • Push your toes into the floor to help keep you stable and maintain your grip.

#10 SIDE BRIDGE

- Lie on one side, with your forearm on the ball and your legs stretched out.

- Place your other arm on your side.

- Raise your hips off the ball. Hold this position for 10 seconds; then lower your hips back down to the ball.

- Repeat for the desired number of repetitions and then switch sides.

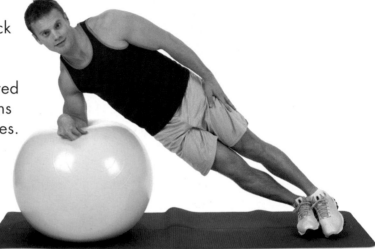

STRENGTH INTENSITY	TONE INTENSITY
3 sets	2 sets
10 reps	15 reps
45 seconds rest between sets	30 seconds rest between sets

HINTS

• Start by lying on your side on the ball. Raise your hips off the ball, and hold this position. • Do not let your hips sag or dip. Keep your upper body aligned with your hips. • Look straight ahead to maintain a neutral spine.

#1 UNI WALL SQUAT

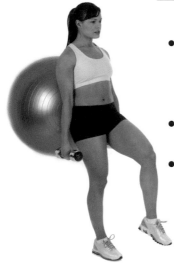

- Start with the ball against the wall at lower-back level. Place your feet ahead of the ball, hip-width apart.

- Hold a dumbbell in each hand.

- Raise one foot off the floor.

- Lower your body down toward the floor, pushing slightly against the ball. Keep one foot in the air, with the leg out front.

- Stop when your thighs are parallel to the floor.

- Return to the starting position and repeat on the other leg.

STRENGTH INTENSITY	TONE INTENSITY
3 sets	2 sets
10 reps	15 reps
45 seconds rest between sets	30 seconds rest between sets

HINTS
- Keep your head up and look straight ahead throughout the movement. Do not look down at the floor or at your feet. • Make sure to keep your standing foot flat on the floor, with your heel down as you move up and down.
- Keep pushing back against the ball throughout the movement.

#2 DUMBBELL PULLOVER

- Lie on your back in a reverse bridge position, with the ball between your shoulder blades and your feet flat on the floor. Keep your hips level with your shoulders.

- Hold one dumbbell in both hands, with your arms fully extended upward and the dumbbell directly over your chest.

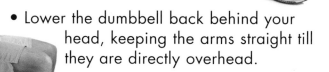

- Lower the dumbbell back behind your head, keeping the arms straight till they are directly overhead.

- Return the dumbbell to the starting position over your chest. Keep your arms completely straight throughout the movement.

STRENGTH INTENSITY	TONE INTENSITY
3 sets	2 sets
10 reps	15 reps
45 seconds rest between sets	30 seconds rest between sets

HINTS

- Keep your hips in line with your shoulders. Do not let them sag or dip.
- You can lower the dumbbell farther behind your head once you feel comfortable with the movement.

#3 ONE-LEG WIDE ROW

- Lie facedown with the ball under your mid-abdomen, your legs stretched out behind, and one foot slightly off the ground.

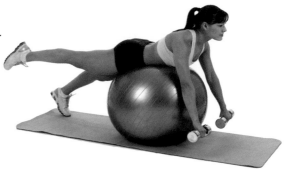

- Hold a dumbbell in each hand with your elbows slightly bent and facing out.

- Raise the dumbbells up, drawing your shoulder blades in and bending your elbows out to the sides.

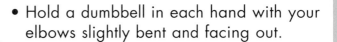

- Lower the dumbbells back toward the floor, extending at the elbows.

- Keep one foot off the ground throughout the movement.

STRENGTH INTENSITY	TONE INTENSITY
3 sets	2 sets
10 reps	15 reps
45 seconds rest between sets	30 seconds rest between sets

HINTS

• Draw your elbows up and out to your sides, not in close. • Look down at the floor to keep your head in line with your spine. • You can move the leg that is off the floor slightly to help you maintain balance on the ball.

#4 UNI BALL LEG CURL

- Lie on your back on the mat, with your heels on the ball and legs extended. Place your hands by your sides.

- Raise your hips off the mat by contracting your abdominals, and raise one foot off the ball, holding your leg up.

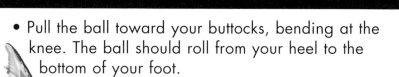

- Pull the ball toward your buttocks, bending at the knee. The ball should roll from your heel to the bottom of your foot.

- Extend your legs, returning the ball to the starting position with your heel back on the ball, keeping the other foot in the air.

- Repeat the exercise, switching the legs.

STRENGTH INTENSITY	TONE INTENSITY
3 sets	2 sets
10 reps	15 reps
45 seconds rest between sets	30 seconds rest between sets

HINTS

- Keep your core and abdominal muscles contracted and maintain a neutral spine throughout the movement. • Push your hands into the floor to help stabilize yourself when raising your hips.
- Keep your head, upper back, and shoulders in contact with the mat throughout the movement.

#5 ONE-LEG FRONT RAISE

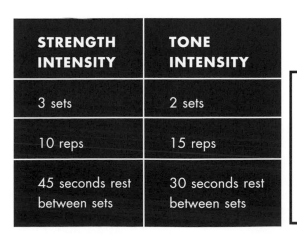

- Sit upright on the ball, with one foot flat on the floor and the other leg extended out in front.

- Hold a dumbbell in each hand, with your palms facing backward and your arms extended by your sides.

- Raise the dumbbells up in front, going just above shoulder level and keeping your arms straight.

- Lower the dumbbells back down to your sides, returning to the starting position. Make sure to go all the way down till the arms are fully extended.

STRENGTH INTENSITY	TONE INTENSITY
3 sets	2 sets
10 reps	15 reps
45 seconds rest between sets	30 seconds rest between sets

HINTS

• Keep your back upright by contracting your core muscles as you raise the dumbbells. • Avoid jerky movements. • You can bend the elbows slightly to avoid too much stress on the shoulder joints.

#6 KNEELING CURL

- Kneel upright on the ball, holding a dumbbell in each hand, with your palms facing forward and your arms extended by your sides.

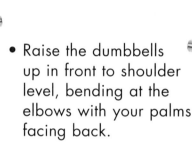

- Raise the dumbbells up in front to shoulder level, bending at the elbows with your palms facing back.

- Return the dumbbells to the starting position at your sides.

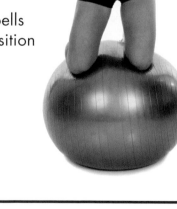

STRENGTH INTENSITY	TONE INTENSITY
3 sets	2 sets
10 reps	15 reps
45 seconds rest between sets	30 seconds rest between sets

HINTS
- Keep your back upright by contracting your core muscles as you raise the dumbbells. • Avoid jerky movements.

#7 DUMBBELL UNI FRENCH PRESS

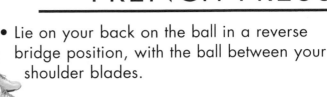

- Lie on your back on the ball in a reverse bridge position, with the ball between your shoulder blades.

- Keep your hips level with your shoulders and your feet flat on the floor.

- Hold a dumbbell in one hand, with your elbow flexed and the weight positioned at the side of your head (by your ear).

- Raise the dumbbell up until your arm is straight and the weight is overhead.

- Lower the dumbbell, bending at the elbow and returning to the starting position. Make sure to go all the way down till the dumbbell is back at the side of your head.

- Repeat for the desired number of repetitions, and then switch sides.

STRENGTH INTENSITY	TONE INTENSITY
3 sets	2 sets
10 reps	15 reps
45 seconds rest between sets	30 seconds rest between sets

HINTS

- Keep your hips in line with your shoulders. Do not let them sag or dip.
- Be careful not to bang the dumbbell against your head as you lift and lower it. • Keep the shoulder steady; movement should occur only at the elbow.

#8 SIDE ROTATION TUCK

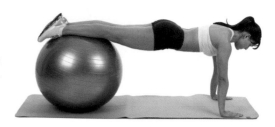

- Start with your hands on the mat directly under your shoulders, with your arms fully extended and your shins on the ball.

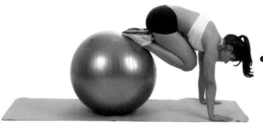

- Drag the ball toward your hands, bending your knees and bringing them to your chest.

- Rotate your lower body to one side, bringing your knees up and to the side.

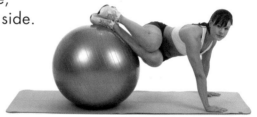

- Extend your knees and straighten your legs, returning the ball to the starting position.

- Repeat the exercise, and rotate to the other side.

STRENGTH INTENSITY	TONE INTENSITY
3 sets	2 sets
10 reps	15 reps
45 seconds rest between sets	30 seconds rest between sets

HINTS

• Keep your hips in line with your shoulders. Do not let them sag or dip. • Look down at the floor to maintain a neutral spin until you rotate; then turn your head to the side you rotate to. • Make sure to keep your hands under your shoulders throughout the movement.

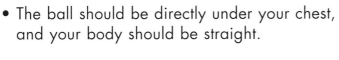

- Start with your hands on the ball, with your arms and your legs extended, and your feet on the floor.

- The ball should be directly under your chest, and your body should be straight.

- Hold this position for 10 seconds, and then lower your body down to lie on the ball.

- Repeat for the desired number of repetitions.

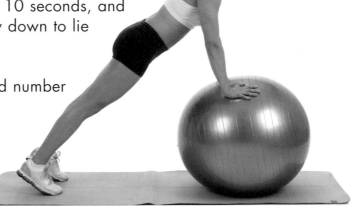

STRENGTH INTENSITY	TONE INTENSITY
3 sets	2 sets
10 reps	15 reps
45 seconds rest between sets	30 seconds rest between sets

HINTS

• Start in a kneeling position, with your hands on the ball. Raise your hips up, and hold your torso in this position throughout the movement. • Make sure to keep your arms fully extended and your hands on top of the ball.

#10 ARM-TO-LEG TRANSFER

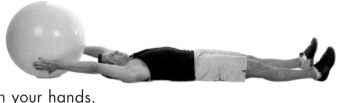

- Lie on your back on the mat, with your legs straight and arms overhead with the ball in your hands.

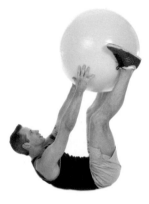

- Simultaneously raise your arms and legs up straight, bringing the ball over your midsection.

- Transfer the ball from your hands to between your feet.

- Lower both your arms and legs, returning to the starting position with the ball between your feet.

- Reverse the movement.

STRENGTH INTENSITY	TONE INTENSITY
3 sets	2 sets
10 reps	15 reps
45 seconds rest between sets	30 seconds rest between sets

HINTS

- Keep your arms and legs straight throughout the movement. • You may put your feet down on the mat at the end of each repetition.

#1 ADDUCTORS 1

- Lie with your back on the mat and the ball in front of you.

- Place your ankles on the ball, with your heels together.

- Gently push your knees away from your body.

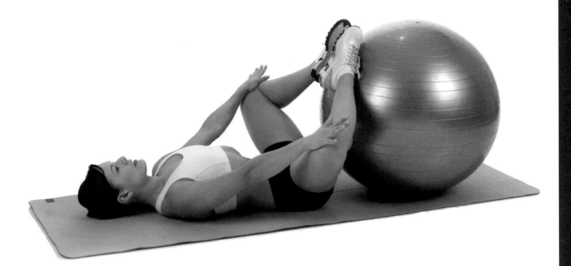

INTENSITY

Hold for 10 seconds.

Repeat 3 times.

#2 GLUTES

- Lie with your back on the mat. Place one leg on the ball with your knee bent. Place the other foot on that knee. Gently push the outside knee away from you.

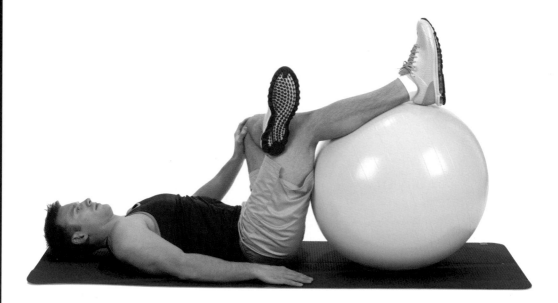

INTENSITY

Hold for 10 seconds.

Repeat 3 times on each leg.

#3 HAMSTRINGS 1

- Lie with your back on the mat. Place one leg on the ball with the knee bent. Keep the other leg straight, and clasp your hands behind your calf or thigh. Slowly pull the leg toward your head.

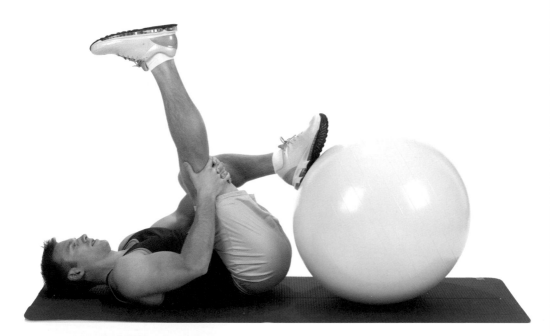

INTENSITY

Hold for 10 seconds.

Repeat 3 times on each leg.

#4 QUADRICEPS 1

- Lie facedown with the ball in your midsection and your feet and hands on the floor. Lift your right leg and grasp your right foot with your right hand, pulling it toward your buttocks.

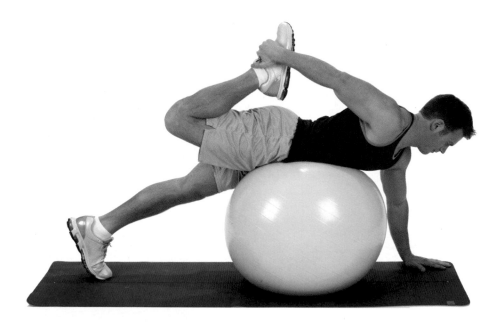

INTENSITY

Hold for 10 seconds.

Repeat 3 times on each leg.

#5 UPPER BACK

- Kneel on the floor with your hands on top of the ball at arm's length.

- Lower your head between your shoulders and arch your back.

- Sit back on your heels.

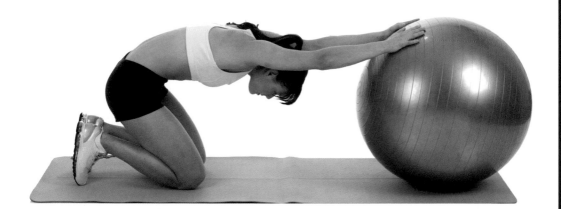

INTENSITY

Hold for 10 seconds.

Repeat 3 times.

#6 BACK

- Lie facedown with the ball in your midsection and your feet and hands on the floor.

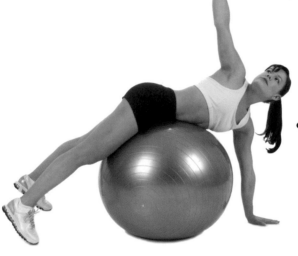

- Raise one arm up, and rotate at your waist. Finish with your arm overhead and directly in line with the other hand on the floor. Look up at the hand overhead.

INTENSITY

Hold for 10 seconds.

Repeat 3 times on each side.

- Lie with your back on the ball and your arms stretched overhead.

- Roll back on the ball so it rests in the middle of your back with your head, shoulders, and arms hanging over the ball. Lower your hands toward the floor.

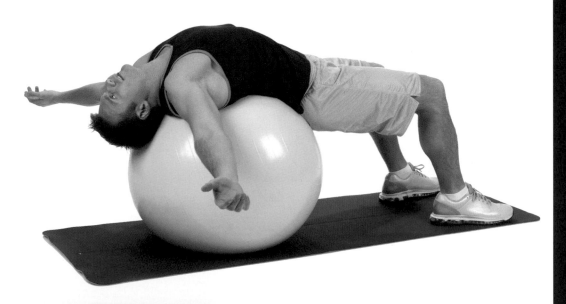

INTENSITY

Hold for 10 seconds.

Repeat 3 times.

#8 LATS 1

- Kneel on the floor, with one hand on top of the ball at arm's length.

- Keep your head down, and look at the floor. Sit back on your heels.

- Lower your shoulder toward the floor until you feel the stretch along the side of your back.

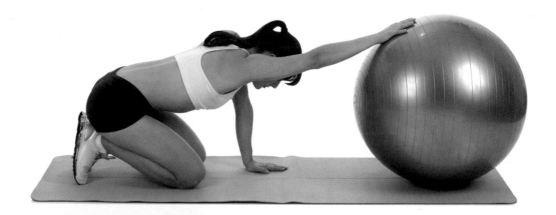

INTENSITY

Hold for 10 seconds.

Repeat 3 times on each side.

#9 SHOULDER

- Kneel on the floor, with the ball in front and one arm resting on top of it. Lift your knees off the floor.

- Lower your upper body toward the ball as you feel a stretch along the back of your shoulder.

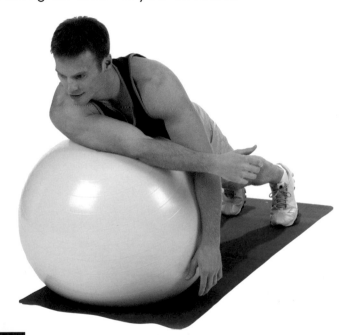

STRETCH SEQUENCE 1

INTENSITY

Hold for 10 seconds.

Repeat 3 times on each side.

#10 TRICEPS

- Sit upright on the ball with one arm behind your head, bent at the elbow.

- Place the other hand on that elbow, and slowly pull it across to the middle of your back.

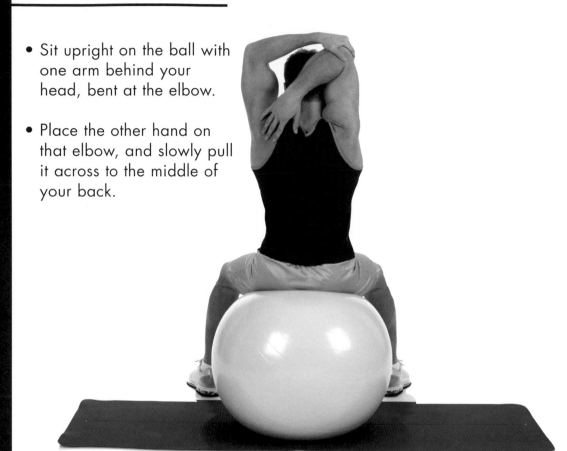

INTENSITY

Hold for 10 seconds.

Repeat 3 times on each arm.

- Stand with the inside ankle of one leg on the ball.

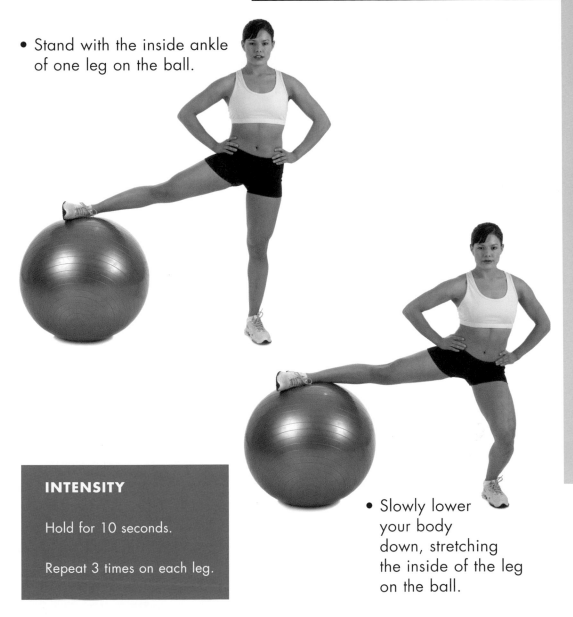

INTENSITY

Hold for 10 seconds.

Repeat 3 times on each leg.

- Slowly lower your body down, stretching the inside of the leg on the ball.

#2 HAMSTRINGS 2

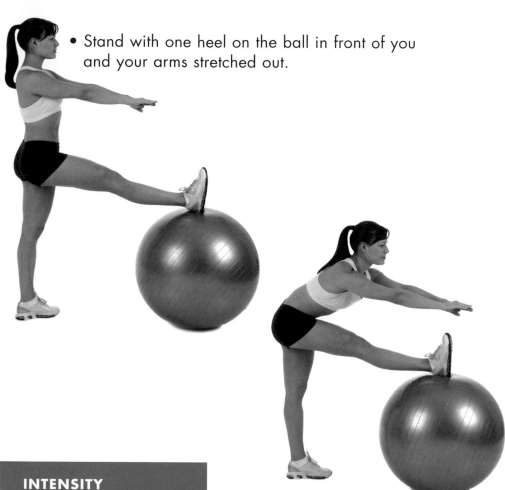

- Stand with one heel on the ball in front of you and your arms stretched out.

INTENSITY

Hold for 10 seconds.

Repeat 3 times on each leg.

- Gently lean forward at the waist, bringing your hands toward your foot.

#3 QUADRICEPS 2

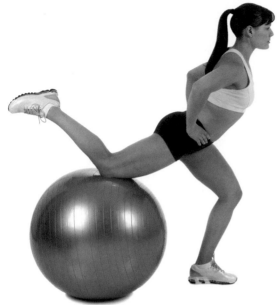

- Stand with one knee on the ball and the other foot in front.

- Gently lean your body weight forward, pushing your knee into the ball.

- For a more intense stretch, hold the ankle of the leg on the ball and pull it toward your buttocks.

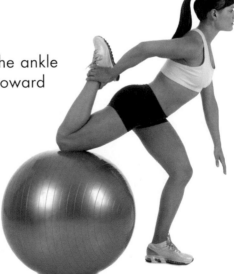

INTENSITY

Hold for 10 seconds.

Repeat 3 times on each leg.

#4 TRICEPS

- Sit upright on the ball with one arm behind your head, bent at the elbow.

- Place the other hand on that elbow, and slowly pull it across to the middle of your back.

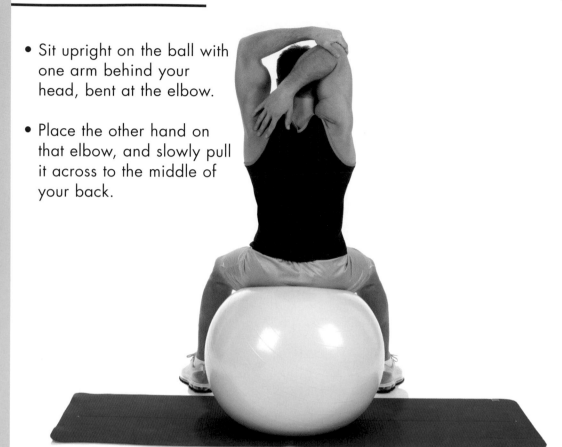

INTENSITY

Hold for 10 seconds.

Repeat 3 times on each arm.

#5 SHOULDER

- Kneel on the floor, with the ball in front and one arm resting on top of it. Lift your knees off the floor.

- Lower your upper body toward the ball as you feel a stretch along the back of your shoulder.

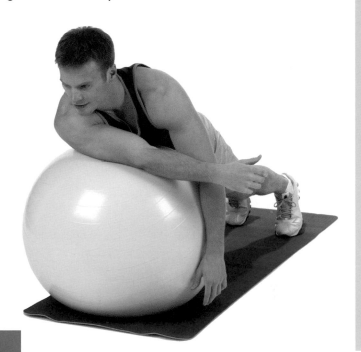

INTENSITY

Hold for 10 seconds.

Repeat 3 times on each side.

#6 CHEST 2

- Kneel on all fours, with the ball to one side of you.

- Place your hand on top of the ball, with your arm extended out.

- Lower your body into a stretch across your upper chest.

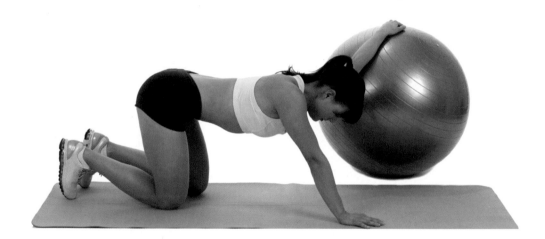

INTENSITY

Hold for 10 seconds.

Repeat 3 times on each side.

#7 UPPER BACK

- Kneel on the floor with your hands on top of the ball at arm's length.

- Lower your head between your shoulders and arch your back.

- Sit back on your heels.

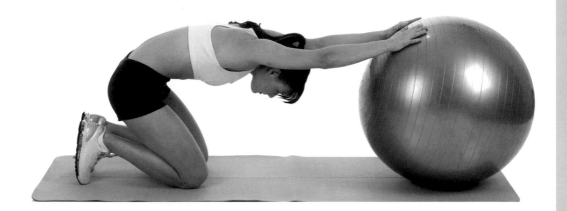

INTENSITY

Hold for 10 seconds.

Repeat 3 times.

#8 LATS 2

- Lie on one side on the ball, with one knee on the mat and the other leg stretched out.

- Arch your body over the ball, and stretch your arms overhead.

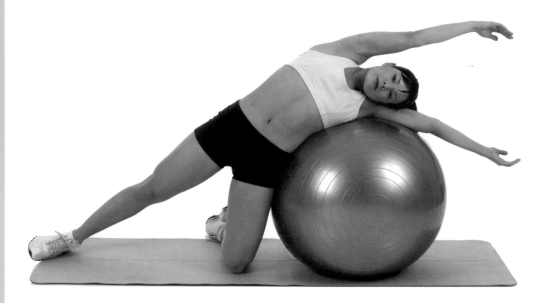

INTENSITY

Hold for 10 seconds.

Repeat 3 times on each side.

- Lie with your back on the mat. Place one leg on the ball with your knee bent. Place the other foot on that knee. Gently push the outside knee away from you.

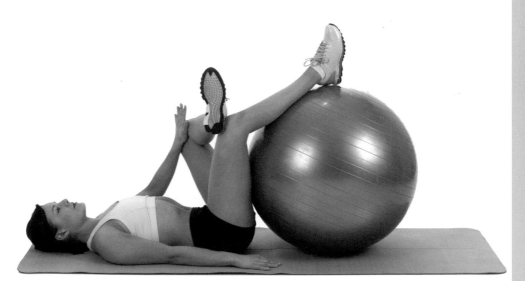

INTENSITY

Hold for 10 seconds.

Repeat 3 times on each leg.

#10 ABDUCTORS

- Lie on your side, with your lower leg on the ball and the other leg behind it.

- Push down on the ball with your leg, and raise your upper body off the mat.

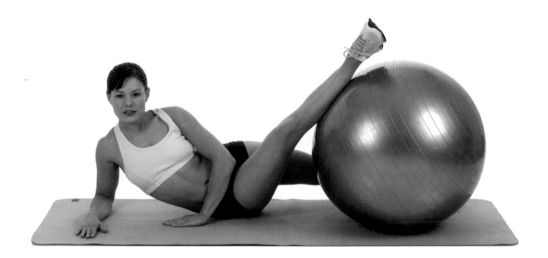

INTENSITY

Hold for 10 seconds.

Repeat 3 times on each leg.

INDEX